HEALTH CARE ISSUES, COSTS AND ACCESS

ACCOUNTABLE CARE ORGANIZATIONS AS A MODEL OF INTEGRATED CARE

HEALTH CARE ISSUES, COSTS AND ACCESS

Additional books in this series can be found on Nova's website under the Series tab.

Additional E-books in this series can be found on Nova's website under the E-book tab.

HEALTH CARE ISSUES, COSTS AND ACCESS

ACCOUNTABLE CARE ORGANIZATIONS AS A MODEL OF INTEGRATED CARE

DANIEL P. DELVECCHIO
EDITOR

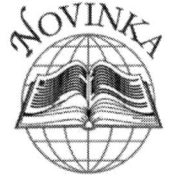

Nova Science Publishers, Inc.
New York

Copyright © 2012 by Nova Science Publishers, Inc.

All rights reserved. No part of this book may be reproduced, stored in a retrieval system or transmitted in any form or by any means: electronic, electrostatic, magnetic, tape, mechanical photocopying, recording or otherwise without the written permission of the Publisher.

For permission to use material from this book please contact us:
Telephone 631-231-7269; Fax 631-231-8175
Web Site: http://www.novapublishers.com

NOTICE TO THE READER

The Publisher has taken reasonable care in the preparation of this book, but makes no expressed or implied warranty of any kind and assumes no responsibility for any errors or omissions. No liability is assumed for incidental or consequential damages in connection with or arising out of information contained in this book. The Publisher shall not be liable for any special, consequential, or exemplary damages resulting, in whole or in part, from the readers' use of, or reliance upon, this material. Any parts of this book based on government reports are so indicated and copyright is claimed for those parts to the extent applicable to compilations of such works.

Independent verification should be sought for any data, advice or recommendations contained in this book. In addition, no responsibility is assumed by the publisher for any injury and/or damage to persons or property arising from any methods, products, instructions, ideas or otherwise contained in this publication.

This publication is designed to provide accurate and authoritative information with regard to the subject matter covered herein. It is sold with the clear understanding that the Publisher is not engaged in rendering legal or any other professional services. If legal or any other expert assistance is required, the services of a competent person should be sought. FROM A DECLARATION OF PARTICIPANTS JOINTLY ADOPTED BY A COMMITTEE OF THE AMERICAN BAR ASSOCIATION AND A COMMITTEE OF PUBLISHERS.

Additional color graphics may be available in the e-book version of this book.

Library of Congress Cataloging-in-Publication Data

ISBN 978-1-62100-120-1

Published by Nova Science Publishers, Inc. † New York

CONTENTS

Preface		vii
Chapter 1	Accountable Care Organizations and the Medicare Shared Savings Program *David Newman*	1
Chapter 2	MEDPAC Comment Letter on Accountable Care Organizations *Medicare Payment Advisory Commission*	65
Chapter Sources		91
Index		93

PREFACE

The provision of health care in the United States has been described as fragmented, with patients seeing multiple providers. Fragmented care has been found to be, among other things, both costly, since provider payments are not linked to performance or outcomes and services can be duplicative, and of lower quality, since providers lack financial incentives to coordinate care. This book examines ACOs as a model of integrated care with a focus on delivery systems such as the Mayo Clinic, Geisinger Health System, Kaiser Permanente and Intermountain Healthcare. While ACOs can be designed with varying features, most models put primary care physicians at the core, along with other providers, and emphasize simultaneously reducing costs and improving quality.

Chapter 1- The provision of health care in the United States has been described as fragmented, with patients seeing multiple unrelated providers. Fragmented care has been found to be, among other things, both costly, since provider payments are not linked to performance or outcomes and services can be duplicative, and of lower quality, since providers lack financial incentives to coordinate care. Section 3022 of the Patient Protection and Affordable Care Act (P.L. 111-148, PPACA), as amended, directs the Secretary of Health and Human Services to implement an integrated care delivery model in Medicare, the Medicare Shared Savings Program, using Accountable Care Organizations (ACOs)—a model of integrated care formulated to reduce costs and improve quality.

Chapter 2- The Medicare Payment Advisory Commission (MedPAC) welcomes the opportunity to comment on the Centers for Medicare and Medicaid Services (CMS) Medicare Shared Savings Program: Accountable Care Organizations proposed rule, published in the April 7, 2011 *Federal*

Register, vol. 76, no. 67, pages 19528 to 19654. The proposed rule addresses many of the myriad issues that will need to be resolved to effectively implement accountable care organizations (ACOs) participating in the Medicare shared savings program under section 3022 of the Patient Protection and Affordable Care Act (PPACA). If structured carefully, a shared savings program for ACOs could present an opportunity to correct some of the undesirable incentives inherent in fee-forservice payment and reward providers who are doing their part to control costs and improve quality. Under the shared savings program the incentives inherent in fee-for-service (FFS) Medicare to increase volume will still be operative and will have to be offset for ACOs to control spending and increase quality. Providers sharing risk with Medicare for cost growth for their patients will strengthen the incentives in the program to control volume and we support moving the program in that direction. The program could also help beneficiaries receive more coordinated care and become more engaged with their care management, particularly if beneficiaries are informed when they are assigned to ACOs, as the authors discuss further in their comments.

In: Accountable Care Organizations as a Model... ISBN: 978-1-62100-120-1
Editors: Daniel P. DelVecchio © 2012 Nova Science Publishers, Inc.

Chapter 1

ACCOUNTABLE CARE ORGANIZATIONS AND THE MEDICARE SHARED SAVINGS PROGRAM

David Newman

SUMMARY

The provision of health care in the United States has been described as fragmented, with patients seeing multiple unrelated providers. Fragmented care has been found to be, among other things, both costly, since provider payments are not linked to performance or outcomes and services can be duplicative, and of lower quality, since providers lack financial incentives to coordinate care. Section 3022 of the Patient Protection and Affordable Care Act (P.L. 111-148, PPACA), as amended, directs the Secretary of Health and Human Services (the "Secretary") to implement an integrated care delivery model in Medicare, the Medicare Shared Savings Program, using Accountable Care Organizations (ACOs)—a model of integrated care formulated to reduce costs and improve quality.

ACOs are modeled on integrated delivery systems such as the Mayo Clinic, Geisinger Health System, Kaiser Permanente, and Intermountain Healthcare. While ACOs can be designed with varying features, most models put primary care physicians at the core, along with other providers, and emphasize simultaneously reducing costs and improving quality. The emphasis is on physicians rather than insurers or hospitals because physicians influence almost 90% of all personal health spending.

In the simplest case, the ACO contracts with payers to be accountable for the entire continuum of care provided to a defined population, and if the costs of care provided are less than targeted amounts, and certain quality measures are achieved, the ACO and the payer will share the savings generated. Under the Medicare Shared Savings Program, the Centers for Medicare & Medicaid Services (CMS) will contract for ACOs to assume responsibility for improving quality of care provided, coordinating care across providers, and reducing the cost of care Medicare beneficiaries receive. If cost and quality targets are met, ACOs will receive a share of any savings realized by CMS. The Congressional Budget Office scored the Medicare Shared Savings Program as reducing Medicare expenditures $4.9 billion in the FY2013 through FY2019 period.

PPACA Section 3022 leaves many of the design features to be determined by the Secretary. On March 31, 2011, the Department of Health and Human Services issued its Notice of Proposed Rulemaking for accountable care organizations. At the same time, the Department of Justice and Federal Trade Commission issued a joint policy statement on ACOs to address antitrust issues. In addition, CMS and the HHS Office of the Inspector General issued a joint statement on the civil monetary penalties law, federal anti-kickback statute, and the physician self-referral law for financial arrangements involving ACOs, and the Internal Revenue Service issued a statement on the participation of tax exempt organizations in ACOs. HHS will accept comments from stakeholders on the NPRM for 60 days and intends to release a final regulation some time afterwards. Appendix A outlines key parts of the proposed regulation, and Appendix B addresses antitrust issues. Appendix C discusses the Pioneer ACO Demonstration "designed for health care organizations and providers that are already experienced in coordinating care for patients across care settings."

The Medicare Shared Savings Program is slated to begin January 1, 2012. While ACOs hold out the prospect of improving care, reducing costs, and raising quality, there are still gaps in knowledge of what existing ACOs have achieved and whether they can be widely replicated. Moreover, there may be unanticipated consequences from encouraging the formation of ACOs, such as further health provider market concentration, that could adversely affect efforts to control overall health costs.

INTRODUCTION

A noted shortcoming in the American health care system is the fragmented care available to most individuals.[1] Fragmented care, where patients see multiple unrelated providers, has been found to be, among other things, both costly, since provider payments are not linked to performance or outcomes and services can be duplicative, and of lower quality, since providers lack financial incentives to coordinate care.[2] Research has suggested that integrated care delivery models can reduce costs and improve quality.[3] Section 3022 of the Patient Protection and Affordable Care Act (P.L. 111-148, PPACA), as amended,[4] directs the Secretary of Health and Human Services (the "Secretary") to implement an integrated care delivery model in Medicare, the Medicare Shared Savings Program, using Accountable Care Organizations (ACOs)—a model of integrated care formulated to reduce costs and improve quality.[5]

While the concept of an ACO is still evolving, Section 1 of this report describes generally what an ACO is, and Section 2 discusses how an ACO may operate. Section 3 describes essential provisions of the Medicare Shared Savings Program created by PPACA. Section 4 explores some of the arguments in favor and against ACOs, and the report concludes with a discussion of the likely impact of Medicare ACOs. The discussion in Sections 1 and 2 focuses on ACOs generally, and Sections 3, 4, and 5 more narrowly focus on the Medicare Shared Savings Program. On March 31, 2011, the Department of Health and Human Services (HHS) issued its Notice of Proposed Rulemaking for ACOs. Appendix A outlines key parts of the proposed regulations, and Appendix B addresses antitrust issues. Appendix C discusses the Pioneer ACO Demonstration that "is designed for health care organizations and providers that are already experienced in coordinating care for patients across care settings."[6]

SECTION 1. WHAT IS AN ACCOUNTABLE CARE ORGANIZATION?

While there are numerous definitions of an accountable care organization, the following captures the essential elements:

ACOs are collaborations that integrate groups of providers, such as physicians (particularly primary care physicians), hospitals, and others around the ability to receive shared-saving bonuses from a payer by achieving measured quality targets and demonstrating real reductions in overall spending growth for a defined population of patients.[7]

The key elements of an ACO, highlighted in the definition, are that

- ACOs bring together and integrate, either actually or virtually, a broad range of providers across care settings;
- they emphasize primary care;
- they can achieve savings for a payer by effectively integrating care across providers;
- providers share with payers in the savings that providers generate;
- the savings are not at the expense of quality;
- providers are responsible for improving quality and reducing costs; and
- improvements are measured across a specified population.

The emphasis is on physicians rather than insurers or hospitals since physicians "control (directly or indirectly) 87% of all personal health spending."[8]

Rationale for Accountable Care Organizations

The rationale for ACOs emerges from the recognition that the current medical system tends to offer fragmented services across providers (an absence of coordinated care), pays for units of service rather than outcomes, and holds no one organization or individual responsible for either the quality or cost of care provided. ACOs are supposed to bring providers together under a single organization and create incentives for them to coordinate care, improve quality, and lower cost.

Although ACOs may contract with any payer (Medicare, Medicaid, or private insurer) to provide services and share in any resulting savings, the consequences for the health care delivery system are assumed to be much broader. Proponents anticipate that ACOs will change both the culture and practice patterns of providers and as these changes are institutionalized, all payers and all patients will benefit from the delivery of higher-quality, lower-cost, and better integrated services.[9]

How Will ACOs Form?

Most ACO proposals assume that *leaders* in the provider community will come together to form an ACO and the ACO will solicit other providers in the community to voluntarily join the ACO to improve the quality of care provided and share in the resulting savings.[10] While this is happening to some extent, the enactment of PPACA has encouraged these efforts as various health care providers seek to position themselves relative to newly formed ACOs.

Since ACOs are perceived as having the potential to alter the influence of primary care physicians, specialist physicians, hospitals, and payers vis-à-vis one another,[11] providers may be motivated to participate in ACOs for a variety of reasons. These include a sincere interest in improving quality of care and reducing costs, a desire to protect their place in the market or to ensure that they have a role in any collective decisions, to share in any cost savings, and to preserve their autonomy.

Existing ACO Models and Are They Replicable

ACOs are modeled on entities seen as quality leaders in health care, such as Kaiser Permanente, the Mayo Clinic, the Cleveland Clinic, and Geisinger Health System.[12] All of these exemplars are highly integrated providers, generally with staff models where physicians are employees of the health care organization. While the above entities are non-profit, there are for-profit models, such as HealthCare Partners Medical Group, with both a staff model and affiliated independent physician association (IPA),[13] and the for-profit Permanente Medical Group that serves Kaiser Permanente. These integrated providers are paid in a variety of ways, including fee-for-service, capitation, and pay-for-performance,[14] and the method of payment does not define the ACO.

It is important to recognize that proponents of ACOs have limited experience replicating the formation and experiences of these integrated providers in more varied organizational environments (see Table 1). The existing models for ACOs, Mayo, Geisinger, and Intermountain, for example, may have had the benefit of physicians self-selecting into a staff model of medical care where physicians are directly employed. New efforts may involve physicians being associated with, but not employed by, the ACO or involve physicians who may not warmly welcome the presence of ACOs but perceive pressure to participate. Such factors may influence the impact of ACOs because providers may be more likely to deviate from directives when they are either not directly employed or feel compelled to participate. Similarly, concern has been expressed that existing examples of ACOs may have unique and potentially nonreplicable characteristics such as an attractive patient population—generally less poor, healthier, and more likely insured.[15]

Table 1. Delivery Systems That Could Become Accountable Care Organizations

Model	Characteristics
Integrated delivery systems	Own hospitals, physician practices, perhaps insurance plan
	Aligned financial incentives
	E-health records, team-based care
Multispecialty group practices	Usually own or have strong affiliation with a hospital
	Contracts with multiple health plans
	History of physician leadership
	Mechanisms for coordinated clinical care
Physician-hospital organizations	Non-employee medical staff
	Function like multispecialty group practices
	Reorganize care delivery for cost-effectiveness
Independent practice associations	Independent physician practices that jointly contract with health plans
	Active in practice redesign, quality improvement
Virtual physician organizations	Small, independent physician practices, often in rural areas
	Led by individual physicians, local medical foundation, or state Medicaid agency
	Structure that provides leadership, infrastructure, resources to help small practices redesign and coordinate care

Source: Health Affairs, *Health Policy Brief: Accountable Care Organizations*, Bethesda, MD, July 27, 2010, http://www.healthaffairs.org/healthpolicybriefs/brief.php?brief_id=20.

SIMILAR ORGANIZATIONAL AND PAYMENT EFFORTS

While the term *accountable care organization* may have a short, recent history, related organizational and payment efforts had been undertaken or were underway at the time of PPACA's enactment. These include the following:

Organizational

Health Maintenance Organizations (HMOs). A model of health care delivery in which an organization provides comprehensive healthcare to enrollees in a specific geographic area using a network of contracted physicians, often with capitated payments, and limits referrals outside the network.[16] An ACO has several features in common with an HMO but the ACO does not limit out-of-network referrals and the insured's relationship to the ACO is far more tenuous than to an HMO.

Medical Homes. "A medical home is an approach to providing primary care where the personal physician has responsibility for the ongoing care of the patient as well as providing and managing the patient's health care needs with other professionals."[17] ACOs are distinguishable from the medical home model which typically emphasizes preventive and primary care or chronic care management and often excludes specialists and hospitals. ACOs typically manage the full continuum of care for its members."[18] The medical home model is compatible with the ACO model and medical homes could affiliate with an ACO just like any other primary care provider or several medical homes could form the nucleus for an ACO.

Organizational and Payment

The Medicare Physician Group Practice Demonstration. "Mandated by the Medicare, Medicaid, and SCHIP Benefits Improvement and Protection Act of 2000 (P.L. 106-554), and started in 2005, creates incentives for physician groups to coordinate the overall care delivered to Medicare patients, rewards them for improving the quality and cost efficiency of health care services, and creates a framework to collaborate with providers to the advantage of Medicare beneficiaries."[19] This demonstration is similar to an ACO model but the demonstration is limited to 10 physician group practices.

The Medicare Health Care Quality Demonstration. Established in 2003 by the Medicare Prescription Drug, Improvement, and Modernization Act (P.L. 108-173, MMA), this demonstration was designed "to examine the extent to which major, multi-faceted changes to traditional Medicare's health delivery and financing systems lead to improvements in the quality of care provided to Medicare beneficiaries, without increasing total program expenditures."[20] Three demonstrations have been funded by the Centers for Medicare & Medicaid Services (CMS) and each is similar in some manner to an ACO—for instance, the Gundersen Lutheran demonstration involves shared savings.[21]

Payment

Pay for Performance. "Pay-for-performance schemes provide financial incentives to health care providers to achieve specified performance/quality targets linking physician pay to the quality of care provided."[22] Unless bonuses are paid out of a withhold pool, they "often add to total costs by paying out incremental bonuses in exchange for meeting certain benchmarks on process measures. ACOs place a much greater emphasis on measuring and rewarding results at the level of a population of patients—not at the level of particular services or episodes that may or may not add up to higher-value care."[23]

Bundled Payments. "Bundled payment systems (also known as "case rates" or "episode-based payment") provide a single payment for all services related to a treatment or condition, possibly spanning multiple providers in multiple settings."[24] ACOs differ from the bundled payment such as the Medicare End-Stage Renal Disease Bundled Payment Demonstration Project To Evaluate Integrated Care Around A Hospitalization, (MMA, § 623(e)) since ACOs seek to "promote efficiency and care on a continuing basis rather than focusing on a single medical episode."[25]

ACOs also have somewhat limited experience in (1) dense urban areas, where insureds have the ability to obtain services more easily from a non-ACO provider, and (2) large rural areas where the ACO may be a virtual entity and there may be a limited sense of shared commitment across providers spread over a large geographic area. Finally, failed similar efforts often recede into the larger health care market and are rarely cited or studied.[26]

Which Providers Are Involved?

While there is general consensus that ACOs seek to integrate a range of providers, there has been an evolution regarding which providers need to be brought into an ACO and whether hospital participation is fundamental to ACOs. While the idealized list of participants from four often-cited ACO proposals is presented below, current thinking is that the composition of ACOs may vary geographically, reflecting local market conditions.[27] However, regardless of which organizations or individuals are involved, analysts have concluded that the effort needs to be provider-led.[28]

- In an early hospital-centric model, from 2007, developed by Elliott Fisher and his colleagues,[29] ACOs were envisioned as a hospital medical staff model in which a hospital and its extended medical staff (those individuals who work within the hospital, those organizations which primarily refer to the hospital, and those providers for whom a majority of their patients are admitted to the hospital), form the basis of an organization responsible for system performance, improving health care quality, and reforming payment.
- In 2008, the Congressional Budget Office (CBO) described a bonus-eligible organization (BEO) model of ACO which was not hospital-centric. The BEO was envisioned to be providers or physicians practicing in groups, networks of discrete physician practices, partnerships or joint ventures between hospitals and physicians, hospitals employing physicians, integrated delivery systems, or community-based coalitions of providers.[30]
- MedPAC described an option for a hospital-centric model of an ACO in 2009 as one that "would consist of primary care physicians, specialists, and at least one hospital. It could be formed from an integrated delivery system, a physician-hospital organization, or an academic medical center."[31]
- By 2010, the earlier Fisher proposal had been transformed from a hospital medical staff model to a non-hospital-centric model that

"involves broad participation and encourages hospitals to participate" but one in which "hospital participation is not an absolute requirement."[32] In this proposal an ACO can include a variety of provider configurations, ranging from integrated delivery systems and primary care medical groups to hospital-based systems and virtual networks of physicians such as independent practice associations.[33]

Five ACO Delivery Models

Table 1 illustrates the various delivery systems that could form the basis for an ACO, however, there is not an archetype organization that one could name associated with each of the model types. In addition to the models listed in Table 1, insurers are now entering the market and evaluating the role they may play within the ACO framework. For instance, both Blue Cross Blue Shield of Massachusetts and Anthem Blue Cross have contracted as ACOs with provider groups in their service regions.[34] In other markets, insurers such as Cigna are working with physician groups to form ACOs.[35]

These five models, and even entities within a model type, are likely to vary by the degree of integration, the role of hospitals, the mix of staff and non-staff physicians, and the sense of a shared commitment to the goals and aspirations of the ACO. In addition, other models may emerge as specialist physicians, who often provide primary care as well as specialty medical services, seek to maintain or improve their market position vis-à-vis other providers and payers.

There are several reasons to believe that hospitals are likely to be integral to ACOs. Given that over 30% of all health care expenditures in 2008 were hospital expenditures,[36] it may be difficult for an ACO to control costs without having a hospital as a participant. In addition, ACOs may require a significant capital investment in their formative years, prior to earning any shared savings, and hospitals are a potential source for these funds.[37] For instance, ACOs are likely, at a minimum, to need to (1) hire staff; (2) acquire unique health information technology, beyond the $22 billion contained in the American Recovery and Reinvestment Act and other investments (P.L. 111-5), that can monitor performance and document improvements in quality across ACO participants; (3) retain legal counsel to contract with the Secretary to participate in the program and to recruit and contract with providers; and (4) develop and disseminate care protocols.[38] Again, those hospitals which are large sophisticated organizations are potentially well positioned to lead these efforts since they can exert some control over a sizable part of health care expenditures and they have capital.

SECTION 2. HOW ARE ACOs SUPPOSED TO WORK?

Just as there are different notions of which providers are essential to an ACO, there are different ideas of how ACOs should work. The discussion below focuses on the simplest arrangements to highlight the features of an ACO and on the several relationships that exist involving ACO and payers (Medicare, Medicaid, and private insurers), ACO and providers, and ACO and insureds (referring generally to either beneficiaries under Medicare or Medicaid or individuals covered by private insurance).

The Relationship between the ACO and Payers

An ACO's principal function is to take responsibility for some or all of the medical care delivered to a population of patients.[39] For an ACO to *take responsibility for a defined population of patients*, it is assumed that the ACO will contract with payers on behalf of its affiliated providers[40] and that the ACO will not get to pick and choose individual patients from within the defined population based on health status. For example, a payer and an ACO may agree that the ACO will take responsibility for all of the payer's insureds who received more than 50% of their primary care from a physician or group of physicians affiliated with the ACO. In this example, the ACO and payer need to agree on the following:

- the historic cost of care for this population (referred to as the "benchmark");
- a formula to calculate anticipated changes in health care costs for this population due to such factors as increases in medical care costs, aging, or changes in health status;
- a targeted savings rate that will trigger payments to the ACO; and
- certain quality measures that the ACO will need to demonstrate have been met.

In this example, the ACO is responsible for *all* medical care, and therefore the ACO would be responsible for coordinating the entire continuum of care from primary to post-acute. To the extent that one entity is responsible for all care, responsibility is unambiguous and care can be fully coordinated.

If actual medical expenditures are less than the benchmark, adjusted for changes in costs, savings exceed the target, and quality measures are met, the ACO, and either directly or indirectly its providers, will share in the savings realized by the payer.

In its simplest form, using Medicare fee-for-service as an example, an ACO would *take responsibility for a defined population of patients*—in this example, all Medicare beneficiaries in the region who received a majority of their primary care in the prior year from providers affiliated with the ACO would be assigned to the ACO. The ACO and Medicare would agree on a benchmark amount of total medical expenditures that reflected historic patterns of spending adjusted by any forecast growth in costs over the agreement period and any other risk adjustments that the ACO and Medicare agreed to, such as age, gender, or the population's health status. In addition, the ACO and Medicare would identify quality measures that either needed to be met or improved upon.[41] Providers would continue to file claims with Medicare on behalf of their patients, and Medicare would pay those claims as if the ACO did not exist. If quality measures were achieved and actual Medicare expenditures were less than anticipated expenditures, by at least the targeted amount, the ACO would be eligible to share in Medicare's savings according to some agreed formula.

In the example above, the ACO and its providers assume no risk related to either the amount that they receive for provided services or the total cost of medical services provided. That is, the ACO is not penalized in any manner if no savings are achieved and providers are paid the full Medicare fee-for-service payment regardless.

There are other payment models that payers and ACOs could adopt that could involve *risk sharing*. In order to include risk sharing in the above example, Medicare could pay providers 95% of the fee-for-service payment and set aside the difference, a 5% withhold, to be paid later, along with a proportion of the shared savings, if quality and expenditure targets were reached. The withhold and savings would be paid to physicians who elected to participate in the ACO, and their share of the savings would be governed by the ACO's internal policies and its agreements with participating physicians. This model creates greater incentives for providers to achieve targeted reductions. Additional risk and incentives can be transferred to the ACO under other models, such as capitation—where a provider is paid a fixed amount per person and is responsible for the cost of all of the care required to be provided.[42]

The ACO model explicitly couples quality and savings and generally requires providers to achieve savings while maintaining or improving quality. For instance, in the CBO's description "[ACOs] would be eligible to receive a bonus only if they met a set of quality performance measures and expenditure saving targets."[43] The linking of quality and savings in this manner may assume that as quality increases, costs decline. However, there are likely to be desirable and costly quality improvements that do not produce savings which may need to be paid for directly. While it is likely that initial quality measures may be relatively limited process-oriented measures, such as compliance with screening and preventive service guidelines, payers are likely to ratchet-up quality improvements and reporting requirements over time if they anticipate a financial return or as validated outcome measures become more readily available.[44]

The Relationship between the ACO and Providers

While there is no requirement that providers affiliate with an ACO, any relationship between an ACO and its providers more than likely will be governed by a contract that specifies the obligations of both parties and how providers share in any savings. There can be multiple ACOs in a community, and conceivably a provider could be a member of one with respect to the practice's Medicare beneficiaries and a member of another with respect to a private insurer's population of insureds.[45] Once a provider affiliates with an ACO, the provider brings all of his or her patients from the defined population (be it Medicare, Medicaid, or a private insurer) to the ACO. It is further assumed that the ACO will be composed of providers that tend to refer to one another (either admitting to the same hospital or referring to a common set of specialists).

To generate shared savings, the ACO, working with its affiliated providers, can, among other things, seek to[46]

- reduce the unnecessary or duplicative use of services;
- develop or adopt existing care protocols to improve coordination of care and management of diseases, increase preventive services, and encourage early diagnosis;
- improve information flows within the ACO;

- promote lower-cost treatment options;
- benefit from economies of scale in the purchase of goods and services;
- reduce preventable emergency department visits and rehospitalizations;
- coordinate the purchase and use of expensive equipment; and
- coordinate the hiring of some specialists to optimize organizational efficiency.

Because an ACO includes a range of providers, some large and potentially influential (such as large medical groups or hospitals) and some smaller and less prominent (such as sole practitioners and small practices), some proposals envision that the ACO will be a separate and distinct legal entity with a shared decision-making structure to ensure that some providers, hospitals, or large practice groups do not dominate internal decision making. Others envision hospitals or physician groups morphing into ACOs.[47]

An unresolved issue at this point is how these shared savings would be distributed to providers within the ACO after it has covered its costs and any return of capital from the organizers. For instance, how much of the savings associated with better primary care/specialist treatment are attributable to the actions of the primary care doctors as compared to the actions of the specialists? In an integrated staff model of health care organization, these potential disputes generally are muted somewhat by the employment relationship and certainty of salary, but in a virtual ACO or less integrated ACO, these divisions are likely to be more contentious. In addition, the ACO may need to decide who can affiliate with it and which cost savings efforts should be pursued. Since these types of decisions touch on earnings and livelihoods, they are also potentially contentious.

The Relationship between the ACOs and Insureds

For proponents of ACOs, one attractive feature of the ACO model is that it does not place a new entity between providers and patients since patients continue to deal with the health care system through their regular sources of care. The provider, in turn, now has a relationship with the ACO, and the ACO has a relationship with the payer. While the ACO is accountable for the total cost of medical care consumed by those for whom it has assumed responsibility, insureds in most ACO models are not constrained by the ACO as to where they get their care (either primary care providers or specialists) or to which hospitals they can go. The ACO is not a closed network or gatekeeper and the insured, in most models, never affirmatively enrolls in the ACO.[48]

As described above, a provider *brings* patients to an ACO when the provider affiliates. Under this model, the insured is essentially automatically enrolled in the ACO as part of the provider affiliating.[49] Since the activities of the ACO do not constrain the choices of the insured (individuals may continue to see any provider), nor do they alter the costs to the insured (there are no differential prices for in-ACO or out-of-ACO providers), the insured has no basis for selecting an ACO or for opting-in or opting-out of an ACO. Moreover, in some models, annual assignment to an ACO takes place retrospectively, based on actual patient-provider associations, so insureds are not in an ACO at the time that they receive services. The retrospective assignment of individuals to an ACO also means that a group of providers will generally not be held responsible for individuals who were not actually affiliated with the ACO because they received most of their care from other providers. In addition, retroactive assignment encourages physicians to treat all patients in a cost-effective manner since they will not know until later whether any particular patient will be assigned to their ACO.

Finally, some suggest that if there are savings to be realized, the consumer should share in these along with the insurer and providers.[50] Others maintain that while the insurer and provider benefit monetarily, consumers benefit from improved quality of care and no further benefit needs to be conferred on the consumer. If consumers insists on receiving a share of savings, or ACOs want to share savings with Medicare beneficiaries, a whole host of issues emerge, including the effect of anti-kickback provisions of Medicare,[51] as well as questions about when beneficiaries should receive payments and the size of payments necessary to align beneficiaries' interests to conform to care protocols or accept lower-cost equivalent quality services. It should be noted that while the Medicare program, through Medicare Advantage, already offers a form of *shared savings* to enrollees when plans reduce cost sharing below the 20% coinsurance generally found in traditional Medicare, the decision as to whether to enroll in Medicare Parts A or B or enroll in a Medicare managed care plan are likely to be made based on a variety of factors. However, sharing savings with Medicare beneficiaries may blur some of the distinctions between ACOs and Medicare Advantage.[52]

SECTION 3. ESSENTIAL PROVISIONS OF § 3022 OF PPACA

Section 3022 of PPACA directs the Secretary to establish a Medicare Shared Savings Program by January 1, 2012. The goals of this section of the law are, in part, to promote the formation of ACOs and "encourage investment in infrastructure and redesigned care processes for high quality and efficient service delivery" (§ 3022(a)(1)).[53] The section applies only to items and services provided under Medicare Part A (hospitalization insurance) and Part B (medical insurance).[54]

PPACA delegates the formulation of many of the details concerning ACOs to the Secretary, including which entities can be an ACO, what requirements will be imposed on ACOs, and what they will need to achieve prior to receiving their share of any shared savings. Section 3022(c), however, does specify:

> The Secretary shall determine an appropriate method to assign Medicare fee-for-service beneficiaries to an ACO based on their utilization of primary care services provided by ACO professionals.

First, the CBO, in its discussion of ACOs (referred to as BEOs prior to the passage of PPACA), estimated that within two years of implementation, 20% of fee-for-service Medicare beneficiaries would be assigned to participating primary care physicians and that 40% would be assigned by 2019.[55] Therefore, while a large number of Medicare beneficiaries are likely to participate in an ACO, the majority, for a variety of reasons, likely will not. Second, the statute directs the Secretary to determine a method to *assign* beneficiaries to ACOs. While the Secretary has the authority to determine a method that permits Medicare beneficiaries to elect to participate, participation does not otherwise appear to be voluntary. Finally, the statute is silent as to whether the assignment is prospective, with Medicare beneficiaries each year being *assigned* for the following year based on last year's patterns of utilization, or retrospective, with Medicare beneficiaries assigned this year for the prior year based on actual patterns of utilization in the prior year. There are advantages and disadvantages to both prospective and retrospective assignment, as discussed below.

The following groups of providers of services or suppliers which have established a mechanism of shared governance are eligible to participate in the Medicare Shared Savings Program:

- Physicians, physician assistants, nurse practitioners, clinical nurse specialists in either group practices or networks of individual practices.
- Partnerships or joint ventures of physicians, physician assistants, nurse practitioners, clinical nurse specialists and hospitals.
- Hospitals employing physicians, physician assistants, nurse practitioners, clinical nurse specialists.
- Other groups of providers of services and suppliers as the Secretary determines.

The requirement that the ACO have a mechanism for shared governance may be an attempt to keep physicians, physician assistants, nurse practitioners, and clinical nurse specialists at the core of the ACO and not have it be dominated by the larger health care providers in a community. Unless addressed by the Secretary, this requirement, however, may be muted by hospitals acquiring primary care practices or health plans adopting staff models that convert physicians, physician assistants, nurse practitioners, or clinical nurse specialists into employees.[56]

In addition, the statute specifies that an ACO must, among other things,

- be accountable for the quality, cost, and overall care of the Medicare fee-for-service beneficiaries assigned to it;
- agree to participate in the program for not less than three years (the "Agreement Period");
- have a formal legal structure that would allow the organization to receive and distribute shared savings to providers of services and suppliers;
- include primary care physicians, physician assistants, nurse practitioners, clinical nurse specialists in sufficient numbers to serve assigned ACO beneficiaries;
- have at least 5,000 fee-for-service Medicare beneficiaries assigned to it;
- establish a leadership and management structure that includes clinical and administrative systems; and
- develop processes that promote evidence based medicine, patient engagement, report on quality and cost measures, and coordinate care.

Providers of services or supplies may be paid in the same manner as other Medicare providers of services or supplies but share in any savings resulting from reduced utilization. PPACA directs the Secretary to establish a *savings requirement*, the amount that the ACO has to reduce average per capita Medicare expenditures by, before the ACO can share in the savings. Actual spending is compared to a benchmark, established by the Secretary, that is based on the "most recent available 3-years of per-beneficiary expenditures for Parts A and B services for Medicare fee-for-service beneficiaries assigned to the ACO." In addition, the benchmark is adjusted by beneficiary characteristics and the projected absolute growth in national per capita expenditures for Parts A and B services (These calculations, as specified in the Notice of Proposed Rulemaking, are explained in Appendix A).

Alternatively, Section 3022 of PPACA, as amended by Section 10307 of the Health Care Education and Reconciliation Act of 2010, P.L. 111-152, authorizes the Secretary, as appropriate, to use a partial capitation model for ACOs that are highly integrated and capable of bearing the risk.[57] In addition, Section 10307 allows the Secretary to use other payment models that improve the quality and efficiency of items or services furnished to Medicare beneficiaries. These alternative payment mechanisms, which may include payment withholding and other forms of risk-sharing, are designed to fund larger financial incentive payments that encourage greater support for ACO initiatives.

SECTION 4. POTENTIAL ADVANTAGES AND LIMITATIONS OF ACOS

Perhaps the most commonly made argument in support of ACOs begins with the premise that the current medical system offers fragmented services across providers (an absence of coordinated care), pays for units of service rather than outcomes, and holds no one organization or individual responsible for either the quality or cost of care provided. The ACO model highlights the need for change that simultaneously alters the financing and delivery of care to align incentives among providers. For instance, there is some evidence to suggest that when fees for services are reduced without altering models of delivery, providers compensate by rendering more units of services and less savings are realized.[58] Similarly, introducing new models of care, such as medical homes, requires changes in payments to encourage providers to implement these new service models. ACO proponents, in essence, say that there is a need to change both care and payments at the same time—we need to bring together Medicare providers of services and supplies, hold them accountable for the services they provide, and reward them for reducing costs and good performance.

A second argument in support of ACOs is that introducing accountability and integration in the health care system may improve access to care; increase efficiency by reducing unnecessary investment, testing, referrals, and medication; improve quality, outcomes, and patient experience; and reduce costs. For ACO proponents, the current system is not sustainable, new models of delivery are needed, and the ACO model is one that many stakeholders appear to be willing to initially embrace.

Another argument in favor of ACOs is that they have been designed to avoid at least three features of health care delivery systems that often concern the public:

- First, a perception that insurance companies are positioned between patients and their health care providers. While health plans owned by insurance companies conceivably could form the basis of an ACO, the ACO model is:

really designed to shift some of the responsibility for costs from health insurers to health care providers. Insurance plans would retain responsibility for insurance risk—the risk that a pool of insureds will need medical care and the severity of their needs while the ACO is responsible for performance risk—the variability in the costs of treating individuals with the same level of disease severity.[59]

> Therefore, within the ACO model the role for insurers is not expanded; however, as noted, insurers may form ACOs.
- Second, a return to the 1980s and that era's model of managed care and health maintenance organizations. Since many Americans prefer to remain outside of organized health plans, particularly seniors in Medicare,[60] the ACO model does not require that Medicare beneficiaries actually join a health plan. Rather, since Medicare beneficiaries will be assigned by a mechanism developed by the Secretary, there is no necessary requirement that beneficiaries be informed that they are part of an ACO and in fact they may never know that they are assigned to a panel.[61]
- Third, closed panels of providers with potentially differential pricing depending on whether a provider is in or out-of-network. Many

Americans have expressed a clear preference for open panels of providers, where they can select their own doctors, without any difference in copayments, rather than closed panels with lower coinsurance when one sees an in-network provider and a higher copayment when one goes out-of-network. While physicians and other health care providers and suppliers may be aware of which providers are in-network and which providers are out-of-network, the Medicare beneficiary assigned to an ACO can pick and choose his or her providers without regard to either a network or differential cost.[62]

ACOs have detractors and ACOs have raised concerns among policy analysts. Randall Brown of Mathematica Policy Research, for instance, has described ACOs as

much like an HMO, but without any real authority. Medicare Advantage plans (HMOs and PPOs) have generally shown themselves to be poor role models for efficiency or delivering higher quality than fee-for-service, despite the appeal of having one entity being responsible for delivery of the full range of health care services to a defined population of patients. Other forms of Medicare Advantage plans, such as private fee-for-service (PFFS) plans, are even less efficient. Furthermore, the logistics of how such a system would or could work anywhere, except perhaps in a small community where physicians are salaried (and therefore have no financial incentive to overuse services), are unclear. As Fisher and colleagues note, there are significant cultural, legal, and practical obstacles to this model. Saving money will require reducing hospital use and unnecessary services provided by physicians; the pie has to shrink. Battle lines will quickly form on which provider's piece will take the biggest hit, and it is unclear who will wield the actual authority in making those decisions. The failure of HMOs to achieve similar promise should be a warning sign, and how accountable health organizations will avoid the same fate is unclear.[63]

While the ACO needs to implement an internal governance structure, as directed by statute, there are concerns on the part of some critics, including University of Virginia professor Jeff Goldsmith, as to whether primary care doctors and specialists practicing in varying arrangements, hospitals, and other providers truly share enough in common to coordinate care and reduce costs.[64] Goldsmith also notes that

- past efforts at forming integrated networks of providers, real or virtual, had the consequence of concentrating provider networks (either hospitals or physicians) that can effectively raise prices when negotiating with private insurers; and
- consumers have repeatedly and strongly expressed their preference for open networks rather than hospital/physician based risk bearing organizations.

A recent study by Berenson, Ginsburg, and Kemper (2010) of the California health care market, a location where ACOs are common, warns that while Medicare may benefit from the introduction of ACOs, the larger health care system could be negatively affected because the consequences of ACOs may not be limited to Medicare. They conclude, based on their study of California, that "if accountable care organizations lead to more integrated provider groups that are able to exert market power in negotiations—both by encouraging providers to join organizations and by expanding the proportion of patients for whom provider groups can negotiate rates—private insurers could wind up paying more, even if care is delivered more efficiently."[65]

A potential limitation of the Medicare Shared Savings Program is that it addresses items and services only under Medicare Parts A and B. Medicare Part D prescription drug benefits in 2010 are estimated to be slightly more than 11% of all Medicare benefits, and ACOs are not initially responsible for these expenditures as part of the Medicare Shared Saving Program. As Crosson has suggested, "it may be useful to consider models in which Part D benefits are incorporated into payment design,"[66] particularly as there may be instances where there is the appearance of cost savings as a result of providers unduly relying on Part D prescription medicines over other forms of care.

SECTION 5. DISCUSSION AND LIKELY IMPACT OF PPACA § 3022

Scope of ACOs and Likely Savings

The CBO scored the Medicare Shared Savings Program as reducing Medicare expenditures $4.9 billion over the FY2013 through FY2019 period.[67] The CBO also estimated, in 2008 and prior to PPACA, that within two years of implementation of an ACO-type program, 20% of fee-for-service Medicare beneficiaries would be assigned to participating primary care physicians and that 40% would be assigned by 2019.[68] The CBO assumes that the savings to Medicare from BEOs would decline over time, in part because as quality improved, more ACOs would be paid their share of any resulting savings. While these projected savings are perhaps an argument in support of ACOs, the size of these savings are also a caution. ACOs have the potential to significantly change the structure of health care markets, with potential unintended consequences, and consolidation around ACOs in the publicly financed part of the health care market may increase costs in the private, non-government, part of the health care market because of consolidation among providers.

Actual Source of Potential Savings

MedPAC maintains that "the financial incentive in a large ACO for physicians to change their individual decisions affecting a single patient are likely to be small."[69] Rather, the real savings from the ACO model are projected to come from the incentives that physicians as a group have to constrain the growth in capacity and growth in the supply of specialists while adopting care protocols and other mechanisms to reduce the growth in Medicare spending.[70] For instance, providers within an ACO may decide to share an imaging machine across entities rather than having each entity purchase its own machine. Since the savings "stem from group rather than individual decisions," ACOs will need a mechanism for collective decision making and the member organizations (physician groups and hospitals) will need to restrict their autonomy and transfer authority to the ACO in order for the ACO to enforce collective decisions. This type of coordinated decision making, across entities, may be difficult to foster.

Limited Experience with Model

An additional concern, as noted earlier, is that the ACO model has a limited track record beyond a handful of integrated health care providers. It remains an open issue as to whether less integrated providers can come together, achieve savings, and internally govern an organization with potentially highly fractured sets of interests. For example, in the start-up phase, which could last several years, ACOs will need to generate operating capital to cover the costs of contracting, developing health information technology (HIT) monitoring and reporting systems, and building compliance programs to report to CMS. This is in addition to any costs associated with implementing care protocols or other cost-reduction or quality improvement efforts. Moreover, ACOs may have some difficulty monitoring which providers are responsible for any savings achieved and avoiding tension over which providers should be compensated and how much, when responsibility may not be clearly attributable. Finally, quality improvements do not always result in savings and some improvements in quality may prove costly.

Informing Beneficiaries

As noted earlier, some proponents and some critics have suggested that Medicare beneficiaries should be informed of their physician's participation in an ACO, and some suggest that Medicare beneficiaries should have the right to either opt-in or opt-out of their physician's ACO panel. Prior notice to a beneficiary implies that assignment to an ACO is prospective rather than retrospective. As a practical matter prospective enrollment, where Medicare beneficiaries are informed of their assignment ahead of time, may be somewhat problematic. First, it requires that CMS base the current year's enrollment on the prior year's utilization, whereas retrospective assignment would allow CMS to assign beneficiaries based on actual utilization. Second, since assignment can change from year-to-year, Medicare may have to inform beneficiaries each year of their assignment and offer to allow beneficiaries to either opt-in or opt-out of the ACO. While an opt-out option would not be dependent on Medicare beneficiaries actually responding, if there is concern about *automatic* enrollment, an opt-in strategy may be more desirable since beneficiaries would not be assigned to an ACO unless they affirmatively indicated their desire to enroll. As with many CMS communications to beneficiaries, while each is intended to inform, these communications may also give rise to potential confusion and increased call-center activity.

Potential Market Consolidation

Returning to the concerns of Berenson, Ginsburg, and Kemper (2010) and Goldsmith, the actual impact of ACOs may depend on how they potentially change local market competition and whether these disparate local interests (including primary care physicians, specialists, hospitals, payers, and other health care professionals including, but not limited to, nurse practitioners, physical therapists, home health care agencies) can work together cooperatively to achieve and share savings. One could find that ACOs offer the Medicare program savings compared to current practices, but that ACOs also raise prices for other payers as providers consolidate under the ACO structure and become potentially more formidable negotiators vis-à-vis other payers.[71] In addition, one may find in some locations ACOs have difficulty reaching agreement regarding which individuals or entities were responsible for generating the savings, and hence should share in any distribution, or that the overhead and program costs of operating the ACO reduce the impact of the limited financial incentives such that some participants drift away from the ACO over time.

Finally, and building on the Berenson et al. (2010) conclusion, since hospitals are likely to be a critical component of any ACO, perhaps essential to controlling costs, hospitals may end up being the prime movers in creating ACOs and the hub around which other providers gravitate.[72] Hospitals may find that once they form an ACO, they have little incentive to assist other ACOs but significant incentives to bring specialists and other providers into the ACO either as staff or affiliates. In addition, in the past, when hospitals have increased their negotiating leverage vis-à-vis payers, they have used their leverage to obtain higher payment rates.[73] It is an unresolved issue, and one that is likely to play out differently in different markets, as to whether hospitals will aim to achieve savings that will need to be shared with their partners.

APPENDIX A. SUMMARY OF HHS DRAFT PROPOSED REGULATIONS

On March 31, 2011, the Department of Health and Human Services (HHS) issued its Notice of Proposed Rulemaking (NPRM) for accountable care organizations.[74] At the same time, the Department of Justice and Federal Trade Commission issued a joint policy statement on ACOs to address antitrust issues. In addition, CMS and the HHS Office of the Inspector General issued a joint statement on the civil monetary penalties (CMP) law, federal anti-kickback statute, and the physician self-referral law for financial arrangements involving ACOs, and the Internal Revenue Service issued a statement on the participation of tax exempt organizations in ACOs. HHS will accept comments from stakeholders on the NPRM for 60 days and will release a final regulation some time afterwards.

Using a question and answer format, this appendix outlines key parts of the proposed regulation. The first two questions are general to the Medicare Shared Savings Program (Shared Savings Program) and the remainder deal with the NPRM.

1. What is the Medicare Shared Savings Program?

Section 3022 of PPACA requires the Secretary to establish the Shared Savings Program. The Shared Savings Program is intended to promote the development of Accountable Care Organizations (ACOs) which will be responsible for a patient population, coordinate items and services under Medicare Parts A and B, and encourage investment in infrastructure and redesigned care processes for high quality and efficient service delivery.

2. What Is an ACO Generally?

ACOs are collaborations that integrate groups of providers, such as physicians (particularly primary care physicians), hospitals, and others (e.g., durable medical equipment suppliers, rehabilitation hospitals, and home health agencies) around the ability to receive shared-saving bonuses from a payer by achieving measured quality targets and demonstrating real reductions in overall spending growth for a defined population of patients.[75]

3. When is the Medicare Shared Saving Program to Begin, How Many ACOs are Likely to Form, and How Many Medicare Beneficiaries are Likely to be Involved with an ACO?

Section 1899(a)(1) of the Social Security Act, as established by PPACA, requires the Secretary to establish the Medicare Shared Savings Program no later than January 1, 2012. While there are no hard estimates of the actual number, in its Notice of Proposed Rulemaking CMS used an estimate of 75 to 150 ACOs for its aggregate cost estimate. Similarly, CMS projections assumed that roughly 1.5 to 4 million Medicare beneficiaries would be assigned to participating ACOs over the first three years.[76]

4. What Is Required of a Medicare ACO?

4.1. Legal Structure

The proposed rule is not prescriptive with respect to the legal structure adopted. Rather, CMS requires only that an ACO certify that it is recognized as a legal entity in the state in which it was established, that it is authorized to conduct business in each state in which it operates, and have a federal tax identification number.[77]

4.2. Shared Governance

In addition to a formal legal structure, ACOs need to establish and maintain a governing body which can define processes that promote evidence based medicine and patient engagement, report on quality and cost measures, and coordinate care. The body must be comprised of ACO participants (at least 75% of the governing board), or their designated representatives, and include *independent* Medicare beneficiary representative(s).

4.3. Primary Care

Medicare beneficiaries are assigned to an ACO according to the historic provision of primary care services by primary care physicians (see paragraph 7). Primary care physicians are those physicians with a primary specialty designation of internal medicine, general practice, family practice, or geriatric medicine. Primary care services mean the set of services identified by the following HCPCS codes:[78] 99201 through 99215, 99304 through 99340, and 99341 through 99350, G0402 (the code for the Welcome to Medicare visit); and G0438 and G0439 (codes for the annual wellness visits).

4.4. Minimum Number of Medicare Beneficiaries

PPACA § 3022(b)(2)(D) requires that an ACO have at least 5,000 Medicare beneficiaries assigned to it. While there were proposals to raise this number, including from MedPAC, the proposed regulations adopt the 5,000 beneficiary minimum. However, since assignment is based on actual prior primary care utilization, not all Medicare beneficiaries seen by an ACO necessarily count toward the 5,000 figure.

5. Who Can Participate in an ACO?

The statute (PPACA § 3022(b)(1)) lists the following groups of providers of services and suppliers as eligible to form an ACO on their own:

i. ACO professionals in group practice arrangements.
ii. Networks of individual practices of ACO professionals.
iii. Partnerships or joint venture arrangements between hospitals and ACO professionals.
iv. Hospitals employing ACO professionals.
v. Such other groups of providers of services and suppliers as the Secretary determines appropriate.

Under section v above, the Secretary proposed to include critical access hospitals (CAHs) that bill for both physician and hospital services.[79]

5.1. What About Critical Access Hospitals (CAHs), Rural Health Centers (RHCs), and Federally Qualified Health Centers (FQHCs)?

While the list in paragraph 5 defines those entities that can participate independently in the program, RHCs, FQHCs, CAHs that bill under the standard method, and other Medicare enrolled providers and suppliers can collaborate with ACOs and share in savings. In fact, there are financial incentives for ACOs to include FQHCs and RHCs as collaborators.

5.2. What about Specialty Practices?

Specialty practices, such as cardiologists or oncologists, can participate in an ACO, however, as noted in paragraph 7, the primary care services delivered by specialists are not used to assign Medicare beneficiaries to an ACO.

6. What Are The Required Elements of an Agreement between CMS and an ACO?

6.1. Terms and Term of Agreement

While there are provisions for terminating an agreement earlier, the statute and proposed regulations require that the ACO commit to a three-year agreement with CMS. In addition, all contracts or arrangements between or among the ACO, ACO participants, ACO providers/suppliers, and other entities providing services related to ACO activities must require compliance with the regulations and the terms of the agreement between CMS and the ACO. The ACO, ACO participants, ACO providers/suppliers, and other entities providing services on behalf of the ACO must also agree to comply with federal criminal law, the False Claims Act, the anti-kickback statute, the civil monetary penalties law, and the physician self-referral law.

6.2. Certifications by ACO

The ACO must certify the accuracy, completeness and truthfulness of its ACO application, the three-year agreement, and all submissions to CMS including quality data or other information that CMS relies on in calculating shared savings payments or losses. This certification is by an individual with the legal authority to bind the ACO. If the data or information is generated by an entity other than the ACO, that entity must certify the accuracy, completeness and truthfulness of the data it generated.

7. How Are Medicare Beneficiaries Assigned to an ACO?

Medicare fee-for-service beneficiaries are assigned to an ACO based on their utilization of primary care services provided by a primary care physician who is an ACO provider/supplier during the performance year for which shared savings are to be determined.

For each ACO, assignment involves a five-stage process:

1. Identify all primary care physicians who were an ACO participant during the performance year.
2. Determine all beneficiaries who received services from primary care physicians in the ACO.
3. Determine the total allowed charges for the primary care services that each of the beneficiaries received from any provider or supplier during the performance year.
4. For each beneficiary, add together the allowed charges for the primary care services provided by the primary care physicians in each ACO.
5. Assign a beneficiary to an ACO if the beneficiary has received a plurality of his or her primary care services, as determined by the sum of allowed charges for those services, from primary care physicians who are ACO participants. The ACO to which they are assigned is the one with which their primary care physician is affiliated.

Medicare beneficiaries enrolled in a Medicare Advantage Plan (Medicare Part C) cannot be enrolled in an ACO.

8. Can an ACO Improve Its Performance by Avoiding Risky Medicare Beneficiaries?

CMS indicated that it intends to use a combination of the methods to identify trends and patterns suggestive of avoidance of at-risk beneficiaries. If CMS determines that an ACO, its ACO participants, any ACO providers/suppliers, or contracted entities performing functions or services on behalf of the ACO are avoiding at-risk beneficiaries, CMS can require the ACO to submit and implement a corrective action plan (CAP). The ACO will not receive any shared savings payments during the probation period, nor will it be eligible to receive shared savings for the performance period attributable to the time the ACO was under the CAP or be eligible to earn shared savings attributable to the time the ACO is under the CAP. The ACO will be re-evaluated during and after the CAP implementation period to determine if the ACO has continued to avoid at-risk beneficiaries. Finally, CMS can terminate its agreement with the ACO if CMS determines that the ACO has continued to avoid at-risk beneficiaries during or after the CAP.

In addition, the costs which the ACO are responsible for are to be risk adjusted to reflect the age and health status, among other things, of its patient population. Moreover, Medicare beneficiaries who did not receive any primary care in the performance period (i.e., very healthy individuals) are not assigned. Finally, it may prove difficult to significantly reduce costs for relatively healthy individuals who receive little care.

9. What Access Will the ACO have to Medicare Beneficiary Data and How Will Personal Data Be Protected?

9.1. What Data will an ACO Have Access to?

ACOs will have access to CMS aggregate data that omits personal identifiers. At the beginning of the agreement period, and each subsequent year, an ACO, upon request, can gain access to the name, date of birth, and Medicare health insurance claim number of each beneficiary that was included in the records used to generate the ACO's benchmark. These data are made available so the ACO can engage in population-based activities relating to improving health or reducing health care costs, protocol development, case management, and care coordination.

CMS will, upon request, provide an ACO with monthly claims data for potentially assigned beneficiaries. These data can be used for purposes of evaluating ACO provider/supplier performance, conducting quality assessment and improvement activities, and conducting population-based activities relating to improved health. As noted in paragraph 10.4 below, Medicare beneficiaries can request that their data not be shared.

The use of identifiers and claims data will be limited to developing processes and engaging in appropriate activities related to coordinating care and improving the quality and efficiency of care that are applied uniformly to all Medicare beneficiaries assigned to the ACO, and these data cannot be used to reduce, limit or restrict care for specific beneficiaries.

9.2. How will Medicare Beneficiary Data Be Protected?

ACOs have to observe all relevant statutory and regulatory provisions regarding the appropriate use of data and the confidentiality and privacy of individually identifiable health information. In addition, ACOs will have to comply with the limitations on the use and disclosure of individually identifiable health information that the HIPAA Privacy Rule places on HIPAA covered entities, as well as all other applicable privacy and confidentiality requirements. Moreover, ACOs will be prohibited from using the data received under the Shared Savings Program for any prohibited use of individually identifiable health information.

If an ACO misuses or discloses data in a manner that violates any applicable statutory or regulatory requirements or that is otherwise non-compliant with the provisions of its data-use agreement with CMS, it will no longer be eligible to receive data and it could potentially be terminated from the Shared Savings Program as well as subject to additional sanctions and penalties.

An ACO will only have access to a beneficiary's claims data if the beneficiary had been seen in the office of a participating primary care physician during the performance year, the beneficiary was informed about how the ACO intends to use the beneficiary's identifiable claims data, and the beneficiary did not exercise the opportunity to opt-out of having his/her claims data shared with the ACO.

10. How are Medicare Beneficiaries Protected?

There are numerous Medicare beneficiary protections incorporated into the proposed regulations. Several of the more salient ones are:

10.1. Medicare Beneficiaries Can Opt-out

The most significant protection afforded Medicare beneficiaries is that an ACO cannot in any way diminish or restrict the right of beneficiaries assigned to an ACO to exercise free choice in determining where to receive health care services.

10.2. Notice

All ACO participants must inform Medicare beneficiaries that they or their ACO providers/suppliers are participating in the ACO. ACO participants must post signs in each of their facilities and provide written notification for beneficiaries about their participation in the Shared Savings Program.

10.3. Marketing Materials

Since historically there have been abuses with the marketing of officially sanctioned Medicare products such as Medigap and Medicare Advantage, ACO marketing materials, and any changes to marketing materials, must be approved by CMS prior to use.

10.4. Beneficiary Claims Data

As noted above, ACOs may have access to the personal data of Medicare beneficiaries. Prior to the ACO requesting Medicare beneficiary claims data from CMS, an ACO must inform beneficiaries that it wants to use their personal health information to coordinate care coordination and improve quality. The ACO has to give beneficiaries a meaningful opportunity to opt-out of having his/her claims information shared with the ACO by supplying beneficiaries with a form allowing them to opt-out of data sharing. The form must be provided to each beneficiary as part of an office visit with a primary care physician.

This requirement will not apply to the initial four data points that CMS will provide to ACOs for individuals in the three-year base data set (Beneficiary Name, Beneficiary DOB, Beneficiary Sex, and Beneficiary health insurance claim number).

10.5. Medicare Beneficiary Representative(s) on Governing Body

As noted above, each ACO governing board must have at least one Medicare beneficiary representative on its governing body ostensibly to represent the interests of Medicare beneficiaries generally.

10.6. CMS Retains Right to Terminate Agreements

CMS may terminate an agreement with an ACO if the ACO, the ACO participants, the ACO providers/suppliers or contracted entities performing services or functions on behalf of the ACO:

(1) Avoid at-risk beneficiaries.
(2) Fail to meet quality performance standards.
(3) Fail to completely and accurately report information or fail to make timely corrections.
(4) Are not in compliance with eligibility requirements or have fallen out of compliance with the requirements because the ACO has undergone material changes that affect the ACO's eligibility to participate in the Shared Savings Program.
(5) Are unable to effectuate any required regulatory changes during the agreement period after given the opportunity for a CAP.
(6) Are not in compliance with requirements to notify beneficiaries of ACO provider/ supplier participation in an ACO.
(7) Engage in material noncompliance, or demonstrates a pattern of noncompliance, with public reporting and other CMS reporting requirements.
(8) Fail to submit an approvable CAP, fail to implement an approved CAP, or fail to demonstrate improved performance after the implementation of a CAP.
(9) Violate the physician self-referral prohibition, civil monetary penalties (CMP) law, Anti-kickback statute, other antifraud and antitrust laws (or enter into a final judgment or other final resolution of antitrust charges by an Antitrust Agency), or any other applicable Medicare laws, rules, or regulations that are relevant to ACO operations.
(10) Submit to CMS false, inaccurate, or incomplete data and/or information, including but not limited to, information provided in the Shared Savings Program application, quality data, financial data, and information regarding the distribution of shared savings.
(11) Use marketing materials or participate in activities or other beneficiary communications, that are subject to review and approval, that have not been approved by CMS.
(12) Fail to maintain an assigned beneficiary population of at least 5,000 beneficiaries.

(13) Fail to offer beneficiaries the option to opt-out of sharing claims information.
(14) Limit or restrict internally compiled beneficiary summary of care or medical records from other providers/suppliers both within and outside of the Shared Savings Program to the extent permitted by law.
(15) Improperly use or disclose claims information received from CMS in violation of the HIPAA Privacy Rule, Medicare Part D Data Rule, Privacy Act, or the data use agreement.
(16) Fail to demonstrate that the ACO has adequate resources in place to repay losses and to maintain those resources for the agreement period.

If an agreement is terminated for any reason before the three-year agreement period is completed, the ACO would forfeit its mandatory 25% withhold of shared savings.

11. Can a Medicare Beneficiary Opt-out of an ACO?

Participation by Medicare beneficiaries is totally voluntary and a Medicare beneficiary can *fully opt-in, partially opt-out, or fully opt-out* of the ACO. The process of *opting in* is essentially passive and the beneficiary simply continues to see the same primary care physician they previously saw. The primary care physician, however, is now a member of the ACO which has assumed responsibility for the patient's complete continuum of care.

Since there is no system of in-network and out-of-network physicians or any differential coinsurance or copayments, a Medicare beneficiary is free to see any physician or specialist they choose to or be admitted to any hospital they want. A Medicare beneficiary would *partially opt-out* whenever they sought services from a provider who was not a member of the ACO.

Since an ACO physician, an ACO hospital, or other ACO provider or supplier cannot opt-out of the ACO, the only method for a Medicare beneficiary to fully opt-out of an ACO would be to seek all Medicare covered services from a non-ACO participating physician, hospital, provider, or supplier.

12. Does a Primary Care Physician That Accepts Medicare Have to Join an ACO?

A Medicare participating primary care physician does not have to join an ACO. However, if a physician joins an ACO, all of the physician's patients who received a plurality of their primary care from that physician would be assigned to the ACO. The ACO model does not allow the physician to selectively register some patients and exclude others.

13. Are Physicians Exclusive to an ACO?

Those primary care physicians whose tax identification number was used to identify Medicare beneficiaries for assignment to an ACO are required to commit to a three-year agreement with CMS and be exclusive to one ACO. ACO participants whose tax identification numbers were not used to identify Medicare beneficiaries for assignment to an ACO are required to commit to a three-year agreement with the ACO. As part of the contracting process, this latter group of ACO participants cannot be required to be exclusive to a single ACO but they can choose to be exclusive.

14. Will ACOs Promote the Use of Electronic Medical Records?

CMS anticipates that at least 50% of an ACO's primary care physicians will be meaningful electronic health record (EHR) users, using certified EHR technology by the start of the ACO's second performance year. CMS retains the right to terminate an ACO if it does not meet this requirement.[80]

15. What Are One-Sided and Two-Sided Payment Models and How Are They to Be Used?

CMS uses the terms *one-sided model* and *two-sided model* to describe two different payment models. In a *one-sided model*, the ACO can share in savings if it achieves both its financial and quality targets. If it fails to achieve its financial target, it is not required to *share* any losses incurred by CMS.[81] In a *two-sided model,* the ACO can share in savings if it achieves both its financial and quality targets but is liable for sharing any losses incurred by CMS if the

ACO does not achieve its financial targets (see paragraphs 17 – 19 and 25 for more detail).

16. How Are Savings Calculated?

There are three steps in calculating payments to ACOs: establishing the historic benchmark on which ACO performance will be judged, computing actual per capita Medicare Part A and B expenditures for the performance year, and then determining savings and shared savings under the applicable one or two-sided model.

16.1. Establishing the Benchmark

To calculate historic Part A and B fee-for-service expenditures for beneficiaries that would have been assigned to the ACO in each of the 3 prior years, CMS will estimate a fixed benchmark that is adjusted for overall growth and beneficiary characteristics, including health status using prospective HCC (hierarchical condition categories) adjustments.[82] The benchmark will then be updated annually during the agreement period, according to statute, based on the absolute amount of growth in national per capita expenditures for Parts A and B services under the original Medicare fee-for-service program. The five steps in calculating the benchmark are:

(1) Calculate annual Parts A and B fee-for-service per capita expenditures for the beneficiaries who would have been assigned for each of the benchmark years (truncating catastrophically large claims).
(2) Determine national growth trend indices and trend them to the third benchmark year (BY3) dollars (BY3 is the most recent benchmark year).
(3) Establish health status indices for each year and adjust these indices so they are restated in BY3 risk.
(4) Compute a three-year risk-and growth-trend adjusted per capita expenditure amount for the patient populations in each of the three benchmark years by combining the initial per capita expenditures for each year with the respective growth and health status indices. The result is risk adjusted per capita expenditures for beneficiaries historically assigned to the ACO in each of the three years used to establish the benchmark stated in BY3 risk and expenditure amounts, and assigned patient populations.

(5) Weight BY3 at 60%, BY2 at 30%, and BY1 at 10% so the benchmark gives greater emphasis to the most recent expenditure and health status of the ACO's assigned beneficiary population.

CMS will update this fixed benchmark by the projected absolute amount of growth in national per capita expenditures for Parts A and B services under the original Medicare fee-for-service program using data from CMS's Office of the Actuary.

Finally, CMS will not take into consideration expenditure increases or decreases under Section 1848 of the Social Security Act related to value-based purchasing programs or the HITECH Act;[83] specifically, the Physician Quality Reporting Initiative, the Electronic prescribing program, or the HITECH Act incentives for eligible professionals.

16.2. Computing Per Capita Medicare Part A and Part B Expenditures

For each performance year,[84] CMS will determine whether the estimated average per capita Medicare expenditures under the ACO for Medicare fee-for-service beneficiaries for Parts A and B services, adjusted for beneficiary characteristics and truncated for large claims, is below the applicable benchmark.

16.3. Determining Savings

Each ACO in the one-sided model will have a minimum savings rate (MSR) based on the number of beneficiaries assigned to the ACO. MSRs generally range from 3.9% to 2.0% with larger ACOs having smaller MSRs,[85] but certain smaller ACOs will be exempt.[86] Each ACO in the two-sided model with have a minimum savings rate of 2%.[87]

In order to qualify for a shared savings payment, the ACO's average per capita Medicare expenditures for the performance year must be below the applicable benchmark by more than its MSR. In addition the ACO must meet the minimum quality performance standards and otherwise maintain its eligibility to participate in the Shared Savings Program.

17. What is the Shared Savings Rate under One-Sided Model?

An ACO can elect to participate in the Medicare Shared Savings Program under the one-sided model but this election only covers their participation in the first two performance years. After year 2, these ACOs will be transitioned to the two-sided model.

An ACO that elected the one-sided model and exceeds its MSR is eligible to share savings net 2% of its benchmark. Some smaller ACOs which meet certain criteria (see paragraph 16.3) will be exempt from the 2% net savings threshold adjustment.

The final sharing rate for an ACO in the one-sided model will be calculated by adding the ACO's earned quality performance sharing rate (see paragraph 22). ACOs under the one-sided model are eligible to receive a maximum of 52.5% of the savings they achieve. A 50% share is dependent on how well they meet quality performance goals. ACOs under the one-sided model may be eligible for an additional 2.5% if they include an FQHC or RHC as an ACO participant depending on the number of assigned Medicare beneficiaries with one or more visit to an RHC or FQHC during the performance year. The amount of shared savings an eligible ACO receives under the one-sided model may not exceed 7.5% of its benchmark.

18. What is the Shared Savings Rate under Two-Sided Model?

For each performance year, CMS determines whether the estimated average per capita Medicare expenditures under the ACO for Medicare fee-for-service beneficiaries for Parts A and B services, adjusted for beneficiary characteristics, is above or below the benchmark. In order to qualify for a shared savings payment under the two-sided model (for shared losses with CMS, see paragraphs 19 and 25.3), an ACO's average per capita Medicare expenditures for the performance year must be below the benchmark, respectively, by more than the minimum savings rate of 2%. In addition, the ACO must meet the minimum quality performance standards established by CMS and otherwise maintain its eligibility to participate in the Shared Savings Program under this part.

An ACO that meets all the requirements for receiving shared savings payments under the two-sided model will receive a payment of up to 60% of all the savings under the benchmark as determined on the basis of its quality performance. In addition, an ACO's shared savings rate may be increased by up to 5.0 percentage points if the ACO includes a RHC or FQHC within its structure, determined on a sliding scale based on the number of assigned Medicare beneficiaries with one or more visit to an RHC or FQHC during the performance year. Finally, the amount of shared savings an eligible ACO receives under the two-sided model may not exceed 10% of its benchmark.

19. How Are Shared Losses Calculated?

To be responsible for sharing losses with the Medicare program, an ACO's average per capita Medicare expenditures for the performance year must be at least 2% above its benchmark costs for the year. ACOs would be responsible for "first dollar shared losses" once the minimum loss rate is exceeded.

The shared loss rate, if expenditures exceed the benchmark, for an ACO under the two-sided model is determined based on the amount of the loss and how well the ACO performed on its quality measures.[88] The amount of shared losses for which an eligible ACO is liable for is capped at 5% in year 1, 7.5% in year 2, and 10% in the third year.

An ACO that elected to start the program in the one-sided model, and hence transitions to the two-sided model in the third year, would be liable for an amount not to exceed 5%.

20. How Will ACOs Demonstrate That They Are Providing Quality Care Generally?

CMS has proposed that ACOs submit data on a set of 65 quality measures and that a quality performance standard be established based on existing Medicare fee-for-service/Medicare Advantage (FFS/MA) data to serve as a quality benchmark against which to consider the ACO's performance on each individual measure.[89] The quality performance standard will be used to calculate a quality performance score for each ACO, which is used to determine whether an ACO will be eligible to share in savings (and to what extent) or remain in the program. During the first performance period (January 1, 2012, through December 31, 2012), the quality performance standard would be set at the complete and accurate reporting of these 65 measures; in the following years, the quality performance standard would be set relative to performance on the measures themselves.

21. Which Quality Measures Are Being Proposed and on What Basis Were These Quality Measures Selected?

The 65 quality of care measures include process, outcome, and patient experience of care measures and span five quality domains: (1) care coordination; (2) patient safety; (3) preventive health; (4) patient/caregiver experience; and (5) at-risk population/frail elderly health. These 65 measures are being proposed for the first performance period only; additional measures for the remaining two years are expected to be determined through rulemaking.

CMS prioritized measures for inclusion in the Shared Savings Program based on a number of criteria, including for example, measures that (1) improve individual health and the health of populations; (2) align with those used in other Medicare incentive programs; (3) are sensitive to administrative burden; and (4) have high impact and/or are cross-cutting.

22. How Are ACO's Quality Performance Scores Calculated and How Will They Be Used?

An ACO would receive a maximum of 2 and a minimum of 0 points for each of the 65 quality measures. Quality points are awarded based on the ACO's performance relative to FFS/MA data. The scale is presented in **Table A-1**.

Table A-1. Sliding Scale Measure Scoring Approach.

ACO Performance Level	Quality Points
90+ percentile FFS/MA Rate or 90+ percent	2.00
80+ percentile FFS/MA Rate or 80+ percent	1.85
70+ percentile FFS/MA Rate or 70+ percent	1.70
60+ percentile FFS/MA Rate or 60+ percent	1.55
50+ percentile FFS/MA Rate or 50+ percent	1.40
40+ percentile FFS/MA Rate or 40+ percent	1.25
30+ percentile FFS/MA Rate or 30+ percent	1.10
< 30 percentile FFS/MA Rate or < 30 percent	0.00

Source: Draft Proposed Regulation, CMS-1345-P, p. 204.

The scores on each of the measures would be added together with each of the five quality domains to calculate a performance score for each domain. The domain performance score will be a percentage of points earned relative to total points possible, with all of the measures weighted equally within each domain. All five domain performance scores would then be averaged to determine the overall quality performance score for the ACO, which is the score that would serve as the basis for calculating the shared savings. All of the domains would be weighted equally, regardless of the number of measures, or characteristics of the measures, in each separate domain. For example, if the ACO was enrolled in the one sided model and achieved 90% of its quality points, the ACO would earn 90% of the 50% of the shared savings it was eligible to earn under the one-sided model.

For the first year, in recognition of the challenges associated with collecting and reporting these quality measures, ACOs will be assumed to meet the quality performance standard if they completely and accurately report on the 65 quality measures.

23. What Will Happen If an ACO Does Not Meet the Quality Performance Standard?

One of two outcomes may occur if an ACO does not meet the quality requirements outlined in the proposed rule: (1) it may be ineligible to share in any savings, and (2) it risks termination from the program. Specifically, an ACO that does not meet the quality performance thresholds for all proposed measures would not be eligible for shared savings, regardless of how much per capita costs were reduced.

If an ACO fails to report on 1 or more of the 65 quality measures, it will be given a chance to submit this data with an explanation for why it failed to do so initially. If the ACO does not submit this data in a timely manner, with no reasonable explanation, then the ACO would be terminated from the program. In addition, if an ACO fails to perform adequately in any one of the five quality domains, the ACO would receive a warning and be given a chance to resubmit its data. However, if the underperformance pattern continues, the ACO may be terminated from the program.

24. How Are Medicare Trust Funds Protected?

24.1. Larger MSR for Small ACOs

In order to avoid sharing savings when the savings are potentially a function of random variation in Medicare spending, CMS has proposed that smaller ACOs, as measured by the number of Medicare beneficiaries enrolled, will have to achieve a higher MSR before being eligible for savings.[90] The larger MSR will protect Medicare trust funds.

24.2. Two-sided Model in Year 3 and Subsequent Years

The requirement that all ACOs transition to a two-sided model in Year 3, and in subsequent years, ensures that ACOs do not only benefit when they perform well but, they will be held accountable when they perform poorly. By requiring that ACOs share in both the up-side and the down-side and recovering money from ACOs when they perform poorly, CMS has sought to protect Medicare trust funds.

24.3. Cap on Total Share of Savings

The ACO upside is capped at 7.5% under the one-sided model and 10% under the two-sided model. If an ACO achieves larger savings, the Medicare trust funds benefit fully beyond these capped amounts.

24.4. Withhold

In both models an ACO's share of savings will be subject to 25% withholding in order to help ensure repayment of any losses to the Medicare program that the ACO is responsible for. The withheld amount will be held until a final reconciliation at the end of the agreement period.

24.5. Reinsurance, Escrow, Surety Bond or Line of Credit

ACOs must obtain reinsurance, place funds in escrow, obtain surety bonds, establish a line of credit as evidenced by a letter of credit that the Medicare program can draw upon, or establish another appropriate repayment mechanism in order to ensure repayment of any losses to the Medicare program in advance of participating in the Shared Savings Program under the two-sided model. On an annual basis the ACO must demonstrate that the repayment mechanism is capable of repaying losses equal to at least 1% of the ACO's per capita expenditures for its assigned beneficiaries from the most recent year data available.

25. An Example of Shared Savings and Losses under the One-Sided and Two-Sided Model

Assume that there are two ACOs, ACO1 is a large ACO, with 60,000 participants, and ACO2 is a small ACO, with 5,000 participants. Each ACO has an assumed benchmark expenditures per Medicare beneficiary of $8,000 per year. Benchmark total spending for ACO1 is $480 million annually and benchmark total spending for ACO2 is $40 million.[91]

25.1. Shared Savings under One Sided Model

An ACO's share of savings under the one-sided model is calculated as:

[Benchmark * (% reduction in Medicare expenditures – MSR) * Quality Score]

If ACO1 fully meets all of its quality performance requirements and achieves a 5% reduction in Medicare expenditures, ACO1 would be entitled to 52.5% of the savings less its minimum savings rate of 2%. Therefore, using the above formula, ACO1 would be entitled to:

[$480,000,000 * (5% - 2%) * 0.525] or $7,560,000.

If ACO2 fully meets all of its quality performance requirements and achieves a 5% reduction in Medicare expenditures, ACO2 would be entitled to 52.5% of the savings less its minimum savings rate of 3.9%. ACO2 has a much larger MSR since it has fewer Medicare beneficiaries assigned to it. Therefore, using the above formula, ACO2 would be entitled to:

[$40,000,000 * (5% - 3.9%) * 0.525] or $231,000.

In both cases, the payment to an ACO is capped under the one-sided model at 7.5% of its benchmark, or $36,000,000 for ACO1 and $3,000,000 for ACO2.

25.2. Shared Savings Under Two Sided Model

An ACO's share of savings under the one-sided model is calculated as:
[Benchmark * % reduction in Medicare expenditures * Quality Score]

Under the two-sided model, if ACO1 fully meets all of its quality performance requirements and achieves a 5% reduction in Medicare expenditures, ACO1 would be entitled to 65% of the savings. Therefore, using the above formula, ACO1 would be entitled to:

[$480,000,000 * (5%) * 0.65] or $15,600,000.

If ACO2 fully meets all of its quality performance requirements and achieves a 5% reduction in Medicare expenditures, ACO2 would be entitled to 65% of the savings also. Under the two-sided model, ACOs share from the first dollar since they also share in any loss. Therefore, using the above formula, ACO2 would be entitled to:

[$40,000,000 * (5%) * 0.65] or $1,300,000.

In both cases, the payment to an ACO is capped under the one-sided model at 10% of its benchmark, or $48,000,000 for ACO1 and $4,000,000 for ACO2.

25.3. Shared Losses under Two Sided Model

An ACO's share of losses is calculated as:
[Benchmark * (the amount Benchmark exceeded less the MLR)] * (1 − Quality Score)]

If ACO1 and ACO2 each exceed their benchmark by 5%, they are liable for their share of any loss that exceeds the 2% minimum loss rate or at most 3% (5% - 2%). However, each ACO's liability is further adjusted as a function of its quality performance. Again, assuming ACO1 fully meets all of its quality performance requirements, it would receive a performance score of 65%. Using the above formula, ACO1's liability to CMS is:

[$480,000,000 * 3% * (1 - 0.65)] or $5,040,000.

In this example, using the formula above, ACO2 would be liable to CMS for:

[$40,000,000 * 3% * (1 - 0.65)] or $420,000.

26. What Is the Withhold and What Function Will It Serve?

CMS will withhold a flat 25% of any performance payment amount due to an ACO until the end of the three-year agreement to encourage ACOs to participate for all three years, protect the Medicare program against losses, and ensure ACOs have an adequate repayment mechanism for any losses.

27. How Will an ACO Know Whether or Not It Is Eligible to Share in Savings?

CMS will notify an ACO in writing whether the ACO qualifies for a shared savings payment, and if so, the amount of the payment due. Similarly, CMS will provide written notification to an ACO of the amount of shared losses, if any, that it must pay to the program. If an ACO has shared losses, the ACO must make payment in full to CMS within 30 days of receipt of notification.

28. How Do ACOs Publicly Report Quality Information?

The proposed rule outlines public reporting requirements for all ACOs. Specifically, it would require that ACOs make public the following information: (1) name and location; (2) primary contact; (3) organizational information including, for example, ACO participants and associated committees and committee leadership; and (4) quality performance standard scores. The ACO would be responsible for making the information public using a standardized format that CMS will promulgate through sub-regulatory guidance.

29. How Will These Quality Efforts Be Aligned with Other Federal Quality Efforts?

In its proposed rule, CMS considers and proposes ways to align federal-level efforts to improve the quality of care between the Shared Savings Program and (1) *existing programs*, and specifically the Physician Quality Reporting System (PQRS) and the Electronic Health Records (EHR) and eRx Incentive Programs; and (2) *quality efforts established by PPACA*, and specifically, the hospital inpatient value-based purchasing program, the Medicaid adult quality measures, and the National Quality Strategy.

With respect to existing programs, ACOs meeting the quality requirements of the Shared Savings Program would also be eligible for the PQRS incentive payment (an ACO would be considered a group practice for purposes of the Medicare Shared Savings Program). While successful participation in the Shared Savings Program does not fulfill the requirements for participation in the EHR Incentive Programs, CMS plans to align the measures used in these two programs and to "leverage the infrastructure and measures specifications being developed for that program."[92] CMS also recognizes that a number of new quality programs were established under PPACA, and notes that the quality domains and categories in each program differ to some degree due to the different constituencies affected.

30. How Much Money Does CMS Anticipate the Medicare Shared Savings Program Will Save?

CMS estimates that federal savings over the first three years from the Medicare Shared Savings Program will range from a low of $170 million (90th percentile) to a high of $960 million (10th percentile). The median estimate is $510 million. The range is dependent on how many ACOs enroll in the one-sided or two-sided model (since these involve different rates of sharing) as well as the actual performance of the ACOs in achieving savings.

31. Are There Any Restrictions On How the ACO Distributes Its Share of the Shared Savings?

There are no restrictions in the proposed regulations on how an ACO can distribute its share of any savings. However, as part of its application, the

ACO needs to describe the criteria it plans to employ for distributing shared savings among its participants, how the proposed plan advances the goals of the Shared Savings Program, and how the plan advances the general aims of better care for individuals, better health for populations, and lower growth in expenditures.

CMS estimates start-up costs and first year operating expenditures for an average ACO at roughly $1,750,000.[93] It is likely that some ACOs may need to pay back some of these funds to those entities that invested in them by funding start-up costs. The regulations do not indicate how CMS will evaluate the shared savings distribution plan or how it will view such payments.

APPENDIX B. ANTITRUST CONSIDERATIONS FOR ACOS

The Patient Protection and Affordable Care Act (PPACA, P.L. 111-148, as amended) encourages health care providers to form ACOs to serve Medicare fee-for-service beneficiaries.[94] Federal agencies and other industry commentators generally recognize that health care providers will be more likely to form ACOs to participate in the CMS program if the ACO structure may also be used for commercially insured patients. As discussed above, the creation and operation of ACOs requires the joint action of market participants. Such joint action may raise antitrust concerns, because "under certain conditions ACOs could reduce competition and harm consumers through higher prices or lower quality of care."[95] As a result, a fact-specific inquiry into each proposed ACO would need to be conducted in order to determine whether the antitrust laws that forbid such activities in restraint of trade would be violated should the ACO be allowed to form.

Though each proposed ACO under the Medicare Shared Savings Program will have different effects on the health care provider market, general principles may be extracted to provide guidance to market participants wishing to participate in the Medicare Shared Savings Program. In order to provide guidance for participation in the Medicare Shared Savings Program, as well as implement the structure for the commercially insured, the Department of Justice (DOJ) and the Federal Trade Commission (FTC) (the Agencies) are working together to create a statement of antitrust policy for the treatment of ACOs that qualify for the CMS Program.[96] The Agencies have issued a proposal for a statement of antitrust enforcement policy regarding ACOs participating in the Medicare Shared Savings Program.

The proposal, if adopted, would outline the basic framework for the treatment of ACOs in the Medicare Shared Savings Program under the antitrust laws, and provide those wishing to form ACOs with guidance as to how to do so without running afoul of the antitrust laws. It would create three tiers of antitrust scrutiny for proposed ACOs that intend to participate in the CMS program. The tiers range from no antitrust review to mandatory antitrust review, depending on the share of the market for the services provided by each participant in the ACO's Primary Service Area (PSA). An ACO's PSA refers to its primary geographic market.[97]

The antitrust laws treat naked price-fixing and market allocation agreements as per se illegal.[98] This means that the courts, through previous experience, have found these types of arrangements to have anticompetitive effects that so outweigh any potential procompetitive benefits that a full analysis of the individual agreement's effects is unnecessary.[99] Instead, the agreement is presumed to be in violation of the antitrust laws. However, that does not mean that market participants cannot collaborate to provide procompetitive benefits that improve services to consumers and lower prices. Certain joint price agreements among health care market participants are evaluated under the rules of reason "if the providers are financially or clinically integrated and the agreement is reasonably necessary to accomplish the procompetitive benefits of integration."[100] A rule of reason analysis evaluates a particular joint action to determine whether it is likely to have substantial anticompetitive effects, and, if it does, whether the procompetitive benefits of the action will likely outweigh those potential antitcompetitive effects, such that the proposed action may yet be permissible despite its antitcompetitive potential.[101]

The FTC and DOJ have long had standards for sufficient financial and clinical integration in the health care market in the Agencies' *Statements of Antitrust Enforcement Policy in Health Care* ("Health Care Statements").[102] However, the Agencies have never had specific criteria for clinical integration. By contrast, PPACA and CMS have listed criteria for eligibility to participate in the Medicare Shared Savings Program, "including (1) a formal legal structure that allows the ACO to receive and distribute payments for shared savings; (2) a leadership and management structure that includes clinical and administrative processes; (3) processes to promote evidence based medicine and patient engagement; (4) reporting on quality and cost measures; and (5) coordinated care of beneficiaries."[103] These criteria have been further elucidated by CMS in the regulations described above.

The DOJ and FTC have determined that these criteria are "broadly consistent with the indicia of clinical integration" in the Health Care Statements as it applies to the Medicare market.[104] The Agencies have also determined that the criteria are likely sufficient for the commercial insurance market. As a result, "the Agencies will provide rule of reason treatment to an ACO if, in the commercial market, the ACO uses the same governance and leadership structure and the same clinical and administrative processes as it uses to qualify" for the Medicare Shared Savings Program.[105] To that end, the Agencies have developed a streamlined method for applying the rule of reason to ACOs that are participating in the Medicare Shared Savings Program. It depends upon ACO participants' share of the market in its PSA. The higher the PSA share, the higher the risk of substantial anticompetitive effects. As a result, depending on an ACO's potential share of the market in its PSA, the ACO may require no initial antitrust review, mandatory antitrust review, or a less rigorous process for those arrangements falling in the middle.

Safety Zone

ACOs that fall into the safety zone have no obligation to notify the Agencies of their formation.[106] The Agencies argue that ACOs falling within the safety zone pose very little risk of competitive concerns and will not challenge their formation, absent "extraordinary circumstances." In order to qualify for the safety zone, "independent ACO participants (e.g., physician group practices) that provide the same service (a 'common service') must have a combined share of 30% or less of each common service in each participant's PSA, wherever two or more participants provide that service to patients from that PSA."[107] Furthermore, hospitals and ambulatory surgery centers must participate on a non-exclusive basis, regardless of their PSA. The safety zone for physicians and other service providers does not differ based on whether the physicians are exclusive or nonexclusive to the ACO, unless they fall within the rural exception or the dominant provider limitation. In other words, physicians and other providers may be exclusive to the ACO, unless an exception applies.

Rural Exception: An ACO may include one physician per specialty from each rural county, but that physician must be *non-exclusive* to the ACO. The ACO will still qualify for the safety zone, even if the inclusion of these physicians "causes the ACO's share of any common service to exceed 30 percent" of the PSA for that service. This is also true for rural hospitals. They may be included in an ACO on a non-exclusive basis without violating the safety zone, even if they would raise the share of the market above 30% for that PSA.

Dominant Provider Limitation: If an ACO has a participant with a 50% share of a service in its PSA that no other ACO participant provides in that PSA (dominant provider), that participant must be non-exclusive to the ACO in order for the ACO to qualify for the safety zone. The ACO, which includes a dominant provider, also cannot require a commercial payer to contract exclusively with the ACO.

The safety zone remains in effect for the duration of an ACO's participation in the Medicare Shared Savings Program.

Mandatory Antitrust Agency Review of ACOs Exceeding the 50 Percent PSA Share Threshold

The proposed CMS regulations will not allow an ACO to participate in the Medicare Shared Savings Program (unless the ACO qualifies for the rural exception discussed above) if its share exceeds 50% "for any common service that two or more independent ACO participants provide to patients in the same PSA, unless, as part of the application process," the proposed ACO provides a letter from either the DOJ or the FTC stating that the agency does not intend to challenge the proposed ACO as violating the antitrust laws.[108] As a result, all ACOs wishing to participate in the Medicare Shared Savings Program must first submit to a mandatory antitrust review by the FTC or DOJ if the ACO will exceed the 50% threshold.

When reviewing these proposed ACOs, the Agencies will consider evidence that the ACOs may provide procompetitive benefits and that the potentially high PSA share may not reflect the ACO's market power. The Agencies have proposed to commit to conducting expedited antitrust reviews for proposed ACOs that exceed the threshold. In order to obtain that review process, the Agencies have also outlined the information that the ACOs would have to provide to the reviewing agency, including all the documents the ACO plans to submit as part of its application for the Medicare Shared Savings Program, documents outlining the ACO's likely impact on prices and its plans to compete in the Medicare and commercial markets, and other information indicating how the ACO will be formed and its potential effects on the market within the PSA.[109] This review process would also be subject to certain other CMS requirements.

ACOs Below the Mandatory Review Threshold, but Outside the Safety Zone

Proposed ACOs that fall into this category would not be required to seek a letter from either the DOJ or the FTC in order to participate in the Medicare Shared Savings Program.[110] Nonetheless, they would appear to pose a higher threat of substantial antitcompetitive effects than those ACOs that fall within the proposed safety zone. Though these ACOs would fall outside the safety zone, they may not be required to undergo scrutiny by the FTC or the DOJ. This will depend upon whether the proposed ACO would provide procompetitive benefits like improving health care quality or reducing prices, rather than increasing prices and reducing consumer choice.

To aid ACOs that would fall into this category, the Agencies have outlined five types of conduct that the Agencies believe ACOs should avoid in order to reduce the likelihood that an ACO will present competitive concerns.[111] First, the ACO should prevent or discourage commercial payers from favoring or directing patients to favor certain providers, including those that do not participate in the ACO. Second, the ACO should not tie sales of its services to the commercial payer's purchase of services outside the ACO and vice versa. Third, the ACO should avoid contracting with providers on an exclusive basis, with an exception for primary care physicians. Fourth, the ACO should not restrict a commercial payer's ability to make available to enrollees information that would aid them in evaluating or selecting providers in a health plan. Lastly, an ACO should avoid sharing among its participants "competitively sensitive pricing or other data that they could use to set prices or other terms for services they provide" outside the ACO.[112]

If the ACO avoids these types of conduct, the Agencies may be less likely to subject the ACO to antitrust scrutiny. While ACOs falling into this category apparently have no obligation to notify the Agencies of their formation, ACOs wishing for greater certainty regarding whether the Agencies plan to challenge the ACO pursuant to the antitrust laws may request an expedited review from one of the Agencies. The review would be similar to that which would be conducted for ACOs exceeding the 50% threshold.[113]

This Proposed Statement of Antitrust Enforcement Policy may be revised. The public has the opportunity to comment on the statement and offer suggestions for changes until May 31, 2011.

APPENDIX C. THE PIONEER ACO DEMONSTRATION PROGRAM

On May 17, 2011, the Centers for Medicare and Medicaid Services (CMS) announced a request for applications to participate in the Pioneer ACO demonstration—an initiative of the Center for Medicare and Medicaid Innovation (CMMI). The Pioneer ACO Demonstration "is designed for health care organizations and providers that are already experienced in coordinating care for patients across care settings. It will allow these provider groups to move more rapidly from a shared savings payment model to a population-based payment model on a track consistent with, but separate from, the Medicare Shared Savings Program."[114] While applications to participate are due by July 18, 2011, and the specifics of the demonstration will in part be determined by the final regulations governing the Medicare Shared Savings Program, this appendix describes some of the similarities and differences between the Medicare Shared Savings Program and the Pioneer ACO demonstration.[115]

Table C-1. Summary Comparison of Medicare Shared Savings Program and Pioneer ACO Demonstration Design Parameters.

Parameter	Medicare Shared Savings Program	Pioneer ACO Demonstration
Authority	The Medicare Shared Savings Program was established by § 3022 of PPACA.	The Pioneer ACO Demonstration is under the CMMI established by § 3021 of PPACA which authorizes the Center to test alternative payment and service delivery models.
Requirement for participation of other purchasers	Not proposed at this time.	Require ACOs to have at least 50% of their total revenues derived from outcomes-based contracts by the end of the second performance period.

Table C-1. (Continued)

Parameter	Medicare Shared Savings Program	Pioneer ACO Demonstration
Expenditure benchmark calculation	Benchmark established using per capita Parts A and B FFS expenditures for beneficiaries historically assigned to the ACO in each of the 3 baseline years, risk adjusted using the prospective HCC model. Benchmark is updated annually by the projected absolute amount of growth in national per capita expenditures for parts A and B services.	Expenditure baseline will be trended forward using a hybrid inflationary factor (50% percentage national average growth, 50% absolute dollar growth).
Expenditure baseline calculation	Establishing the benchmark includes weighting the 3 years of the benchmark: BY3 at 60%, BY2 at 30%, BY1 at 10%.	Similar to Shared Savings Program Notice of Proposed Rule Making (NPRM) – Except that Pioneer ACOs will have additional months of lag between the most recent baseline year of 2010 and the start of the first performance period (anticipated to be in the third or fourth quarter of 2011).
Length of agreement	3-yr agreement .	Minimum of three performance periods (slightly longer than 3 years), with two one-year optional extensions.
Core payment arrangement	Track 1: One-sided model for Yr 1 and Yr 2 automatically transitions to two-sided model in Yr 3. Track 2 - Two sided model for all 3 years.	One arrangement with escalating shared savings and shared losses then transition to population- based payment in Yr 3. In addition, solicit suggestions of alternatives from applicants. Synthesize and distill suggestions. Offer all Pioneers choice of 2 final arrangements.

Table C-1. (Continued)

Parameter	Medicare Shared Savings Program	Pioneer ACO Demonstration
Timing of alignment	Retrospective using claims from the performance year, with prospective sharing of population data.	Prospective or retrospective. Prospective using 3 yr prior claims (with time lag only for the first performance period), or retrospective using claims from the performance period and potentially claims from prior years.
Minimum number of aligned beneficiaries	5,000.	15,000 (5,000 for rural).
Beneficiary attestation	Not proposed at this time.	Alignment of beneficiaries who attest ACO as their primary care coordinator and who are newly eligible for Medicare or newly disenrolled from a Medicare Advantage plan after accrual of at least 12 months of FFS experience in the preceding calendar year, or newly relocated to the ACO's market who already have at least 12 months of FFS experience (but added to expenditure calculations only in the subsequent performance period).
Beneficiary choice regarding sharing beneficiary identifiable data	Beneficiaries may decline sharing of identifi-able claims data after notification during an office visit with a primary care physician in the ACO	Beneficiaries would have 30 days for opt-out before data sharing begins; can opt out to stop data sharing at any point thereafter. Process repeats with each performance period.
ACO legal status requirements	Requires ACO to be a legal entity with its own TIN [tax identification number], recognized and authorized under state law	Identical to Shared Savings Program NPRM.

Table C-1. (Continued)

Parameter	Medicare Shared Savings Program	Pioneer ACO Demonstration
Alignment algorithm	Plurality of allowed charges for primary care physicians (internal medicine, general practice, family practice, and geriatric medicine) participating in the ACO.	Pioneer Model would allow non-MD PCPs [primary care physicians], allow alignment with certain specialists if beneficiary has PCP services totaling <10% of all evaluation and management services.
Rapid data feedback	Monthly minimum necessary beneficiary identifiable data, quarterly and annual aggregated reports, baseline ACO spending performance and utilization data.	Pioneer Model will offer monthly financial reports, historical claims data, and may develop additional reports based on input from Pioneer ACOs, but will provide similar quarterly and annual aggregate reports to ACOs.
Legal and regulatory guidance	Separate guidance issued by FTC, DOJ, and IRS. OIG and CMS issued joint guidance on the application of antifraud laws.	Pioneer ACO Model will apply rules consistent with the guidance issued by FTC, DOJ and IRS. On fraud and abuse issues, OIG and CMS expect to apply consistent principles to the consideration of fraud and abuse waiver designs for all ACO programs and models in the Medicare program.
Minimum Savings Rate [MSR]/overspending percentages	MSR based on number of assigned beneficiaries under the one-sided model. Flat rate of 2% under the two-sided model.	Flat rate of 1%.
Governance structure requirements	Legal entity, shared governance, governance body with representative membership, where ACO participants have at least 75% control, and includes patient representation.	Similar to Shared Savings Program with an additional requirement that the board include a consumer advocate.

Table C-1. (Continued)

Parameter	Medicare Shared Savings Program	Pioneer ACO Demonstration
Required HIT capabilities	By the second performance year 50% of an ACO's PCPs are meaningfully using certified EHR [electronic health record] technology as defined in the HITECH Act and subsequent Medicare regulations by start of the second performance year.	Identical to Shared Savings Program NPRM.
Patient centeredness criteria	Eligibility criteria & beneficiary experience of care survey.	Identical to Shared Savings Program NPRM.
Performance metrics	65 measures, developed with input from experts & stakeholders, aligned with CMS and HHS quality initiatives and private sector efforts, set a high bar for quality performance and performance on patient experience measures.	Identical to Shared Savings Program regulation.
Primary care capability	Sufficient to assign at least 5,000 beneficiaries.	Similar, except to be consistent with 15,000 beneficiary minimum (minus the beneficiaries who may be aligned through specialists).
Linkage between quality score and shared savings/ loss percentages (including pay for reporting in the first performance period)	Increased savings for higher quality performance; decreased losses for higher quality.	Similar to proposed Shared Savings Program regulation for the two-sided model except that shared losses will be subject to a minimum in certain cases.

Source: Centers for Medicare & Medicaid Services, http://innovations.cms.gov/wp-content/uploads/2011/05/Pioneer-ACO-RFA.pdf and Congressional Research Service analysis.

ACKNOWLEDGMENTS

The author would like to thank Kathleen Ruane for authoring Appendix B, Antitrust Considerations for ACOs, and Amanda Sarata for authoring sections of Appendix A on quality and quality measurement.

End Notes

[1] Alain C. Enthoven, "Integrated Delivery Systems: The Cure for Fragmentation," *The American Journal of Managed Care*, vol. 15, no. 10 (December 2009), pp. S284-S290.

[2] Institute of Medicine, "Aligning Payment Policies with Quality Improvement," in *Crossing the Quality Chasm: A New Health System for the 21st Century* (Washington, DC: The National Academies Press, 2001), pp. 181-195.

[3] Laura A. Tollen, *Physician Organization in Relation to Quality and Efficiency of Care: A Synthesis of Recent Literature*, The Commonwealth Fund, Commonwealth Fund pub. no. 1121, April 2008. http://www.commonwealthfund.org/~/media/Files/Publications/Fund%20Report/2008/Apr/Physician%20Organization%20in%20Relation%20to%20Quality%20and%20Efficiency%20of%20Care%20%20A%20Synthesis%20of%20Recent%20Literatu/Tollen_physician_org_quality_efficiency_1121%20pdf.pdf.

[4] Hereinafter, PPACA will refer to PPACA as amended.

[5] Section 2706 of PPACA authorized a four-year Medicaid and CHIP pediatric ACO demonstration starting January 1, 2012. This report does not address the Pediatric ACO Demonstration.

[6] http://innovations.cms.gov/areas-of-focus/seamless-and-coordinated-care-models/pioneer-aco/.

[7] This definition is a modified version of that developed in Aaron McKethan, Mark McClellan, Elliott Fisher et al., *Moving from Volume-Driven Medicine Toward Accountable Care*, Health Affairs, Health Affairs Blog, August 20, 2009, http://www.healthaffairs.org/blog.

[8] Lawton Robert Burns and Ralph W. Muller, "Hospital-Physician Collaboration: Landscape of Economic Integration and Impact on Clinical Integration," *Milbank Quarterly*, vol. 86, no. 3 (2008), p. 377, citing A. Sager and D. Socolar 2005. *Health Costs Absorb One-Quarter of Economic Growth 2000-2005*. Boston: Boston University School of Public Health.

[9] A recent study by the Commonwealth Fund comparing the U.S. health care system to other countries found that the U.S. system underperformed in part due to poor performance managing chronic care and coordinating care—two areas directly addressed by ACOs according to proponents. Karen Davis, Cathy Schoen, and Kristof Stremikis, *Mirror, Mirror on the Wall: How the Performance of the U.S. Health Care System Compares Internationally, 2010 Update*, The Commonwealth Fund, Washington, DC, June 23, 2010, http://www.commonwealthfund.org/Content/Publications/ Fund-Reports/2010/Jun/Mirror-Mirror-Update.aspx?page=all.

[10] For instance, in New Hampshire, the New Hampshire Citizens Health Initiative in 2010 issued an *Accountable Care Organization Call for Proposal* "to health care leaders in the state to

ascertain interest and commitment to improving the value of health care delivery systems." http://www.unh.edu/chi/media/documents/NH-ACO-Call-for-Proposal.pdf.

[11] Arlene Weintraub, "Community Hospitals Scramble To Survive, Stay Independent," *USA Today*, September 9, 2010, Web edition.

[12] See Atul Gawande, "The Cost Conundrum: What A Texas Town Can Teach Us About Health Care," *The New Yorker*, June 1, 2009, and Alain C. Enthoven, "Integrated Delivery Systems: The Cure for Fragmentation," *The American Journal of Managed Care*, vol. 15, no. 10 (December 2009), pp. S284-S290.

[13] A staff model is one in which the physicians are employees of the medical group. An independent physician group, in this context, involves the medical group contracting with independent physicians to provide services on behalf of the group as independent contractors rather than as employees.

[14] There are a variety of mechanisms used to pay for medical services, including some hybrid models. In fee-for service, a provider generally bills uniquely for each service provided. In a capitated model, a provider is paid a single amount for assuming responsibility for some or all of the care an individual or population may require. Pay-for-performance models (P4P) seek to compensate providers for better outcomes rather than additional services.

[15] Alex MacGillis and Rob Stein, "Is the Mayo Clinic a Model or a Mirage? Jury is Still Out," *The Washington Post*, September 20, 2009, Web edition.

[16] Modified definition from Stephen M. Shortell, Lawrence P. Casalino, and Elliott Fisher, *Implementing Accountable Care Organizations*, Berkeley Center on Health, Economic and Family Security, Berkeley, CA, May 2010, p. 16. http://www.law.berkeley.edu/files/chefs/Implementing_ACOs_May_2010.pdf.

[17] Rural Assistance Center, *Medical Homes Frequently Asked Questions: What is a Medical Home?* http://www.raconline.org/info_guides/medicalhomes/faq.php.

[18] Baker & Hostetler, "Health Law Update," June 24, 2010, http://www.bakerlaw.com/health.

[19] https://www.cms.gov/DemoProjectsEvalRpts/downloads/PGP_Fact_Sheet.pdf, July 21, 2010.

[20] https://www.cms.gov/DemoProjectsEvalRpts/downloads/MMA646_IHIE_Fact_Sheet.pdf, July 21, 2010.

[21] Descriptions of the three demonstrations can be found at http://www.cms.gov/demoprojectsevalrpts/md/itemdetail.asp?filterType=none&filterByDID=99&sortByDID=3&sortOrder=descending&itemID=CMS023618&intNumPerPage=10 for

[22] Tim Doran and Catherine Fullwood, "Pay for performance: Is it the best way to improve control of hypertension? "*Current Hypertension Reports*, vol. 9, no. 5 (October 2007).

[23] Aaron McKethan, Mark McClellan, Elliott Fisher et al., *Moving from Volume-Driven Medicine Toward Accountable Care*, Health Affairs, Health Affairs Blog, August 20, 2009, http://www.healthaffairs.org/blog.

[24] Rand Corporation, *Overview of Bundled Payment*, Policy Options, http://www.randcompare.org/policy-options/ bundled-payment.

[25] Baker & Hostetler, "Health Law Update," June 24, 2010, http://www.bakerlaw.com/health-law-update-june-24-2010.

[26] For instance, see Liz Freeman, "HMA to buy Cleveland Clinic," *Naples Daily News*, January 25, 2006, Web edition and Liz Freeman, "Physicians apply for medical privileges," *Naples Daily News*, February 27, 2006, Web edition.

[27] See Kelly Devers and Robert Berenson, *Can Accountable Care Organizations Improve the Value of Health Care by Solving the Cost and Quality Quandaries?* Robert Wood Johnson Foundation and Urban Institute, Washington, DC, October 2009, p. 3, http://rwjf.org/files/research/acobrieffinal.pdf and Alain C. Enthoven, "Integrated Delivery Systems: The Cure for Fragmentation," *The American Journal of Managed Care*, vol. 15, no. 10 (December 2009), p 289.

[28] As discussed in section 4 below, PPACA specifies that physicians, physician assistants, nurse practitioners, clinical nurse specialists (collectively referred to as "ACO professionals") in either group practices or networks of individual practices; partnerships or joint ventures of

ACO professionals and hospitals; hospitals employing ACO professionals; and other groups of providers of services and suppliers as the Secretary determines are eligible to participate as ACOs.

[29] See Elliott S. Fisher, Douglas O. Staiger, Julie P.W. Bynum et al., "Creating Accountable Care Organizations: The Extended Hospital Staff Model," *Health Affairs*, vol. 26, no. 1 (January/February 2007) W44-W57. Elliott Fisher, Director of the Center for Health Policy Research at the Dartmouth Medical School, and Mark McClellan, former CMS administrator, formed the Dartmouth-Brookings Partnership and the Accountable Care Organization learning Collaborative. Dr. Fisher is generally credited with the term "accountable care organization."

[30] Congressional Budget Office (CBO), *Budget Options Volume I; Health Care*, Washington, DC, December 2008, pp. 72-74, http://www.cbo.gov/ftpdocs/99xx/doc9925/12-18-HealthOptions.pdf.

[31] See Medicare Payment Advisory Commission, "Report to Congress: Improving Incentives in the Medicare Program," Washington, DC, June 2009, p. 39, http://www.medpac.gov/documents/Jun09_EntireReport.pdf.

[32] Mark McClellan, Aaron N. McKethan, Julie L. Lewis et al., "A National Strategy to Put Accountable Care into Practice," *Health Affairs*, vol. 29, no. 5 (May 2010), p. 983.

[33] An independent physician association is a group of independent physicians that contract with one or more insurers to provide medical care for a population of insureds.

[34] Ken Terry, "'Accountable Care Organizations' Promise Better Medicine for Lower Cost - If They Work," *BNET The CBS Business Network*, June 11, 2010, http://www.bnet.com/blog/healthcare-business/-8220accountable-care-organizations-8221-promise-better-medicine-for-lower-cost-8212-if-they-work/1432.

[35] Leigh Page, "12 Points on Private Payor CIGNA's Plans for ACOs ," *Becker's Hospital Review*, September 30, 2010. http://www.beckershospitalreview.com/hospital-physician-relationships/12-points-on-private-payor-cignas-plans-for-acos.html.

[36] https://www.cms.gov/NationalHealthExpendData/downloads/tables.pdf, Table 2.

[37] The potential capital costs are sufficiently large that Miller has suggested that ACOs may require loans or front-loaded payment arrangements to deal with these investments. Harold D. Miller, *How to Create Accountable Care Organizations*, Center for Healthcare Quality and Payment Reform, Pittsburgh, PA, September 7, 2009, p. 35. http://www.createhealthcarevalue.com/data/blog/HowtoCreateAccountableCareOrganizations1.pdf.

[38] Some proponents anticipate that ACOs may have costs marketing to and communicating with patients of its affiliated providers. Others have suggested that ACOs be paid for demonstrating "sustained savings" (see the comments of Dr. Stuart at the September 13, 2010, MedPAC Public Meeting, http://www.medpac.gov/transcripts/913-914MedPACfinal.pdf, p. 72). The more regulations require ACOs to do up front (marketing or compensating insureds) or the longer any process defers bonus payments, the more difficult it may be to form ACOs.

[39] The more care the ACO is responsible for, the less likely the ACO is in the position to shift costs beyond its areas of responsibility. Hence, many ACO descriptions refer to the "entire continuum of care."

[40] Kaiser Permanente, and other insurer based models, would be exceptions since the payer and ACO may be the same entity.

[41] There are competing perspectives on whether ACOs should be required to meet absolute quality objectives or demonstrate improvement relative to their own past performance. See "Negotiations Over ACO Rule Heat Up As Quality Coalition Urges Changes" *InsideHealthPolicy.com Daily News*, August 19, 2010, http://insidehealthpolicy.com/201008192049189/Health-Daily-News/Daily-News/negotiations-over-aco-rule-heat-up-as-quality-coalition-urges-changes/menu-id-212.html.

[42] MedPAC has analyzed issues associated with risk sharing and the implications of varying sizes of ACOs. See Medicare Payment Advisory Commission, *Transcript of Public Meeting*, September 13, 2010, http://www.medpac.gov/ transcripts/913-914MedPACfinal.pdf.

[43] See Congressional Budget Office (CBO), *Budget Options Volume I; Health Care*, Washington, DC, December 2008, pp. 72-74, http://www.cbo.gov/ftpdocs/99xx/doc9925/12-18-HealthOptions.pdf, for the CBO's calculation of shared savings.

[44] Some proponents have suggested that one area where quality can readily be monitored and improved is rehospitalizations. While not all claims associated with rehospitalizations are avoidable and there are costs to avoiding a rehospitalization, "the cost to Medicare of unplanned rehospitalizations in 2004 was $17.4 billion." If ACOs had greater responsibility for a longer interval surrounding hospitalizations, from 4 days prior to a hospitalization to 30 days following a hospitalization, the interests of physicians and hospitals could be better aligned and the two may be better able to coordinate post-acute care and reduce the high rate of rehospitalization (19.6% within 30 days) among Medicare beneficiaries. See CRS Report R40972, *Medicare Hospital Readmissions: Issues, Policy Options and PPACA*, by Julie Stone.

[45] There is insufficient experience to know the optimal size for an ACO or the optimal number of ACOs in any region. MedPAC and others have suggested that an ACO should have more than 5,000 Medicare enrollees to reduce the random variation in year to year health care expenditures in any pool of patients that might complicate the calculation of both a baseline level of expenditures and actual expenditures. Hussey et al., ("Episode-Based Performance Measurement and Payment: Making It A Reality," *Health Affairs*, vol. 28, no. 5, p. 1406-1417) suggest that 5,000 may be appropriate to hold organizations accountable for more common conditions but larger numbers would be required to hold organizations accountable for rarer events such as heart failure. MedPAC analysis suggests that 5,000 Medicare enrollees may not be adequate to avoid mistakenly paying some ACOs for reductions in costs that occurred by chance (see David Glass and Jeff Stensland, *Medicare Shared Savings Program for ACOs*, Medicare Payment Advisory Commission, prepared for the September 13, 2010, public meeting, Washington, DC).

[46] Some ACO activities may have antitrust or other legal and regulatory constraints, which are beyond the scope of this report.

[47] Section 3022(b) provides that the ACO have a "formal legal structure that would allow the organization to receive and distribute payments for shared savings."

[48] In the private sector, the insured is still governed by the insurance contract between the insurer and the insured, and this contract may impose constraints such as differential coinsurance depending on whether an insured sees an in-network or out-of-network provider.

[49] PPACA provides that the Secretary shall determine the process for assigning Medicare beneficiaries to an ACO and the draft regulations provide for retrospective assignment (see the Appendix). During the public MedPAC meetings, several MedPAC commissioners have spoken in favor of giving Medicare beneficiaries the right to opt-out of participating in any Medicare ACO that their provider may choose to join.

[50] Jeff Goldsmith, "The Accountable Care Organization: Not ready for Prime Time," *Health Affairs Blog*, http://healthaffairs.org/blog/2009/08/17/the-accountable-care-organization-not-ready-for-prime-time/print/, August 17, 2009.

[51] "Under the federal anti-kickback statute, it is a felony for a person to knowingly and willfully offer, pay, solicit, or receive anything of value (i.e., 'remuneration') in return for a referral or to induce generation of business reimbursable under a federal health care program. The statute prohibits both the offer or payment of remuneration for patient referrals, as well as the offer or payment of anything of value in return for purchasing, leasing, ordering, or arranging for, or recommending the purchase, lease, or ordering of any item or service that is reimbursable by a federal health care program." See CRS Report RS22743, *Health Care Fraud and Abuse Laws Affecting Medicare and Medicaid: An Overview*, by Jennifer Staman.

⁵² If Medicare ACOs are required to enroll Medicare beneficiaries into an ACO (see Section 5) and in some manner potentially share savings with beneficiaries, the line between ACOs and Medicare Advantage plans may erode and CMS may want to consider whether ACOs need to be subject to regulations similar to those applicable to Medicare Advantage plans.

⁵³ ACOs are not limited to Medicare and can offer their services to other payers, including Medicaid and private insurers, that may be willing to contract with them.

⁵⁴ The Affordable Health Care for America Act, H.R. 3962, would have allowed the Secretary to include Medicare Part D services, if appropriate.

⁵⁵ Note that the CBO assumed that the program would begin January 1, 2013, whereas PPACA directs the Secretary to establish the shared savings program by January 1, 2012, hence the timeframe for the CBO estimates does not align perfectly to PPACA, nor does it incorporate all of the other elements contained in PPACA.

⁵⁶ Noam N. Levey, "Healthcare law has more doctors teaming up," *Los Angeles Times*, July 28, 2010, http://www.latimes.com/news/health/healthcare/la-na-health-doctors-20100728, 0,2722731.story.

⁵⁷ In a partial capitation model, a part of a provider's compensation is a function of a fixed-flat rate per patient and a part is based on another payment mechanism.

⁵⁸ See for example, Suzanne M. Codespote, William J. London, and John D. Shatto, Estimated Volume-and-Intensity Response to a Price Change for Physicians' Services. Memorandum to Richard S. Foster, Chief Actuary, Centers for Medicare & Medicaid Services, 1998, http://proquest.umi.com/pqdweb?index=6&did=1970670331&SrchMode=3&sid=1&Fmt=6&VInst=PROD&VType=PQD&RQT=309&VName=PQD&TS=1281357481&clientId=45714&aid=1. For a contrasting perspective, see Jack Hadley, James Reschovsky, Catherine Corey et al., "Medicare Fees and the Volume of Physicians' Services," Inquiry, vol. 46, no. 4 (Winter), p. 372–390.

⁵⁹ Harold D. Miller, *How to Create Accountable Care Organizations*, Center for Healthcare Quality and Payment Reform, Pittsburgh, PA, September 7, 2009, http://www.createhealthcarevalue.com/data/blog/HowtoCreateAccountableCareOrganizations1.pdf.

⁶⁰ In 2010, about 24% of Medicare beneficiaries have elected to join a Medicare Advantage plan. http://www.kff.org/ medicare/upload/2052-14.pdf.

⁶¹ The House Tri-Committee's proposal, the America's Affordable Health Choices Act of 2009, required that beneficiaries be informed of their assignment to an ACO, whereas the Senate Finance Committee's America's Healthy Future Act of 2009 did not stipulate that beneficiaries be informed. See Kelly Devers and Robert Berenson, *Can Accountable Care Organizations Improve the Value of Health Care by Solving the Cost and Quality Quandaries?* Robert Wood Johnson Foundation and Urban Institute, Washington, DC, October 2009, p. 6, http://rwjf.org/files/ research/acobrieffinal.pdf.

⁶² While a private insurer could offer different incentives for insureds to use in-network providers, these incentives would come from the insurer and not the ACO. It may be the case that a private insurer employing an ACO to control costs and improve quality would coordinate its efforts such that the ACO network and in-network providers were similar.

⁶³ Randall Brown, *Strategies for Reining in Medicare Spending Through Delivery System Reforms: Assessing the Evidence and Opportunities*, The Henry J. Kaiser Family Foundation, Washington, DC, September 2009, p. 5. http://www.kff.org/medicare/upload/7984.pdf.

⁶⁴ Jeff Goldsmith, "The Accountable Care Organization: Not ready for Prime Time," *Health Affairs Blog*, http://healthaffairs.org/blog/2009/08/17/the-accountable-care-organization-not-ready-for-prime-time/print/, August 17, 2009. Also note the fractious environment between the hospital and physician group at City of Hope National Medical Center has been held out as "a harbinger of things to come under health care reform." Patrick J. McDonnell, "City of Hope's reorganization plan creates rift with doctors group," *Los Angeles Times*,

September 22, 2010, http://www.latimes.com/news/local/la-me-city-hope-20100922,0,5277469.

[65] Robert A. Berenson, Paul B. Ginsburg, and Nicole Kemper, "Unchecked Provider Clout in California Foreshadows Challenges to Health Reform," *Health Affairs*, vol. 29, no. 4 (April 2010), p. 700.

[66] Francis J. Crosson, "Medicare: The Place to Start Delivery System Reform," *Health Affairs*, Web Exclusive January 27,. 2009, pp. W232-W234.

[67] Letter from Douglas W. Elmendorf, Director, Congressional Budget Office, to Honorable Nancy Pelosi, Speaker, House of Representatives, March 20, 2010, http://www.cbo.gov/ftpdocs/113xx/doc11379/AmendReconProp.pdf.

[68] Note that the CBO assumed that the program would begin January 1, 2013, whereas PPACA directs the Secretary to establish the shared savings program by January 1, 2012, hence the timeframe for the CBO estimates does not align perfectly to PPACA.

[69] Medicare Payment Advisory Commission, "Report to Congress: Improving Incentives in the Medicare Program," Washington, DC, June 2009, p. 51, http://www.medpac.gov/documents/Jun09_EntireReport.pdf.

[70] Medicare Payment Advisory Commission, "Report to Congress: Improving Incentives in the Medicare Program," Washington, DC, June 2009, pp. 49-52, http://www.medpac.gov/documents/Jun09_EntireReport.pdf.

[71] CMS has acknowledged potential unintended consequences in the market for health care. http://news.bna.com/hdln/HDLNWB/split_display.adp?fedfid=17792088&vname=hcenotallissues&fn=17792088&jd=a0c4d7x7v4&split=0.

[72] Jeff Goldsmith has suggested that the ACO legislation has prompted hospital consolidation already, http://news.bna.com/hdln/HDLNWB/split_display.adp?fedfid=17792088&vname=hcenotallissues&fn=17792088&jd= a0c4d7x7v4&split=0.

[73] Kelly J. Devers, Lawrence P. Casalino, Liza S. Rudell et al., "Hospitals' Negotiating Leverage with Health Plans: How and Why Has It Changed," *Health Services Research*, vol. 38, no. 1 (February 2003), pp. 419-446.

[74] The complete NPRM can be found at http://www.gpo.gov/fdsys/pkg/FR-2011-04-07/pdf/2011-7880.pdf.

[75] This definition is a modified version of that developed in Aaron McKethan, Mark McClellan, and Elliott Fisher, et al., *Moving from Volume-Driven Medicine Toward Accountable Care*, Health Affairs, Health Affairs Blog, August 20, 2009. http://www.healthaffairs.org/blog.

[76] Department of Health and Human Service, "Medicare Shared Savings Program: Accountable Care Organizations," 76 *Federal Register* 19633, April 7, 2011.

[77] This last requirement appears to preclude contractual joint ventures that do not involve a unique independent entity being created.

[78] HCPCS codes are used by CMS and unique codes are assigned to medical tasks and procedures.

[79] Some critical access hospitals (CAHs) bill under the so-called *standard method* and do not submit claims with information on individual practitioners, or the type of health professional (for example, physician, PA, NP), that provided a specific service. These CAH cannot be an ACO participant.

[80] Meaningful use is defined in the American Recovery and Reinvestment Act of 2009 (P.L. 111-5) as: (1) demonstrating to the satisfaction of the Secretary the use of certified EHR technology in a meaningful manner (including e-prescribing), including for the purpose of exchanging electronic health information to improve health care quality; and (2) using such certified EHR technology to report clinical quality measures, as selected by the Secretary.

[81] The term *losses* actually refers to Medicare expenditures that exceed a benchmark rate, risk-adjusted, that also reflects growth in national per capital expenditures for Medicare Parts A and B.

[82] The HCC methodology uses claims data to predict future medical expenses for each beneficiary.
[83] For more information, see CRS Report R40161, *The Health Information Technology for Economic and Clinical Health (HITECH) Act*, by C. Stephen Redhead.
[84] The agreement between an ACO and CMS is for three years, initially starting January 1, 2112. Each calendar year is a performance year.
[85] The MSR declines with ACO size to ensure that CMS does not pay ACO for savings that occur by chance.
[86] CMS proposes to exempt ACOs with less than 10,000 assigned beneficiaries in the most recent year for which CMS has complete claims data (for instance, 2012 for 2014 program participation) and that meet one of the following: 1) the ACO is comprised only of ACO professionals in group practice arrangements or networks of individual practices of ACO professionals; 2) at least 75 % of the ACO's assigned beneficiaries reside in counties outside a Metropolitan Statistical Area (MSA); 3) at least 50% of the ACO's assigned beneficiaries were assigned to the ACO on the basis of primary care services received from a Method II CAH; or 4) at least 50% of the beneficiaries assigned to the ACO had at least one encounter with an ACO participant FQHC and/or RHC in the most recent year for which CMS has complete claims data.
[87] All ACOs electing to participate in the program under the two-sided model, regardless of size, have the same MSR. The Medicare Program is protected from down-side risk by having ACOs share in any losses.
[88] The formula is [(1-(Final Sharing Rate)) * Amount over the Benchmark] where an ACO which achieved all of its quality measures would have a final sharing rate of .60. In addition, the amount over the benchmark has to be greater than 2%.
[89] The sections on quality and quality measures were written by Amanda Sarata, Domestic Social Policy Division, Congressional Research Service.
[90] The need for a larger MSR is addressed in MedPAC's response to CMS's Request for Information Regarding Accountable Care Organizations and the Medicare Shared Savings Program, published in the *Federal Register*, vol. 75, no. 221, pages 70165 to 70166.
[91] The fact pattern for this example is from PriceWaterhouseCoopers http://pwchealth.com/cgi-local/hregister.cgi?link= reg/stalking-the-aco-unicorn.pdf, registration required.
[92] 76 FED. REG. 19592 (April 7, 2011).
[93] The American Hospital Association estimated the start-up costs to establish a hospital-centric ACO, assuming a 200 bed hospital, 80 primary care physicians, and 150 specialists at $5.3 million with on-going annual costs of $6.3 million. See American Hospital Association and McManis Consulting, *The Work Ahead; Activities and Costs to Develop an Accountable Care Organization*, American Hospital Association, Washington, DC, April 2011, http://www.aha.org/ aha/content/2011/pdf/aco-white-paper-cost-dev-aco.pdf.
[94] This appendix was written by Kathleen Ruane, American Law Division, Congressional Research Service.
[95] *Proposed Statement of Antitrust Enforcement Policy Regarding Accountable Care Organization Participation in the Medicare Shared Savings Program*, 76 Fed. Reg. 21894, 21895 (2011) [hereinafter *Proposed Statement for ACOs*].
[96] *Id.*
[97] PSA is the lowest number of contiguous postal zip codes from which participants draw at least 75% of their patients. Guidance on calculating PSA appears at 76 Fed. Reg. 21899.
[98] Arizona v. Maricopa County, 457 U.S. 332 (1982) (finding a joint pricing agreement between competing physicians to be a per se violation of the antitrust laws).
[99] Northern Pacific Railroad Co. v. United States, 356 U.S. 1, 5 (1957). *See also*, White Motor Co. v. United States, 372 U.S. 253, 263 (1963); United States v. Topco Associates, 405 U.S. 596, 607-08 (1972); Broadcast Music, Inc. v. Columbia Broadcasting System, Inc., 441 U.S. 1, 9-10 (1979); Arizona v. Maricopa County Medical Society, 457 U.S. 332, 344 (1982).

[100] *Proposed Statement for ACOs*, 76 Fed. Reg. at 21895.
[101] *Id.*
[102] Dep't of Justice & Fed. Trade Comm'n Statements of Antitrust Enforcement Policy in Health Care (1996) [hereinafter Health Care Statements] available at http://www.ftc.gov/bc/healthcare/industryguide/policy.
[103] *Proposed Statement for ACOs*, 76 Fed. Reg. at 21896.
[104] *Id.*
[105] *Id.*
[106] *Id.* at 21897.
[107] *Id.*
[108] *Id.* at 21897.
[109] *Id.* at 21898.
[110] *Id.*
[111] *Id.*
[112] *Id.*
[113] *Id.* at 21899.
[114] http://innovations.cms.gov/areas-of-focus/seamless-and-coordinated-care-models/pioneer-aco/.
[115] The complete Request for Application can be found at http://innovations.cms.gov/wp-content/uploads/2011/05/ Pioneer-ACO-RFA.pdf.

In: Accountable Care Organizations as a Model... ISBN: 978-1-62100-120-1
Editors: Daniel P. DelVecchio © 2011 Nova Science Publishers, Inc.

Chapter 2

MEDPAC COMMENT LETTER ON ACCOUNTABLE CARE ORGANIZATIONS

Medicare Payment Advisory Commission

Dr. Donald M. Berwick
Administrator
Centers for Medicare & Medicaid Services
200 Independence Avenue, SW
Suite 314-G
Washington, DC 20201

RE: File code CMS-1345-P

Dear Dr. Berwick:

The Medicare Payment Advisory Commission (MedPAC) welcomes the opportunity to comment on the Centers for Medicare and Medicaid Services (CMS) Medicare Shared Savings Program: Accountable Care Organizations proposed rule, published in the April 7, 2011 *Federal Register*, vol. 76, no. 67, pages 19528 to 19654. The proposed rule addresses many of the myriad issues that will need to be resolved to effectively implement accountable care organizations (ACOs) participating in the Medicare shared savings program under section 3022 of the Patient Protection and Affordable Care Act (PPACA). If structured carefully, a shared savings program for ACOs could present an opportunity to correct some of the undesirable incentives inherent in fee-forservice payment and reward providers who are doing their part to control costs and improve quality. Under the shared savings program the incentives inherent in fee-for-service (FFS) Medicare to increase volume will still be operative and will have to be offset for ACOs to control spending and increase quality. Providers sharing risk with Medicare for cost growth for their patients will strengthen the incentives in the program to control volume and we support moving the program in that direction. The program could also help beneficiaries receive more coordinated care and become more engaged with their care management, particularly if beneficiaries are informed when they are assigned to ACOs, as we discuss further in our comments.

The proposed rule thoughtfully addresses many aspects of the program and discusses the pros and cons of different approaches. Among them are the specific qualifications ACOs must demonstrate, such as a clear management and leadership structure, clear arrangements to assure the continuum of patient care, and commitments to evidence-based and patient-centered care delivery. It also addresses assignment of beneficiaries to ACOs, quality, the shared savings models, coordination with other agencies concerning waivers and antitrust, and overlap with other CMS shared savings initiatives. The proposed rule addresses these issues and asks for comments on specific matters. In this letter, we comment on the following six areas that we think will be crucial to the program's success:

- Prospective assignment of Medicare beneficiaries so that they can be informed of their assignment to ACOs and become fully engaged with improved care management.
- Risk adjustment of the ACO population.
- Focusing on a set of quality measures that reflect the outcomes ACOs are designed to achieve.
- Assessing benchmarks, spending and savings at some form of standardized prices.
- Allowing assignment based on primary care provided in RHC, FQHCs, and by non- physician practitioners.
- Extending the one-sided risk model while protecting against random variation.

Our comments are intended to simplify the program and reduce uncertainty and administrative burden for providers who may wish to form ACOs. Providers may be reluctant to commit time and money to reorganize the delivery system to better coordinate care and improve quality, if rewards are uncertain and difficult to calculate. Our comments on assignment, risk adjustment, quality, and how to reduce initial administrative costs may help address those concerns. However, even if these changes were implemented in the final rule, the number of ACOs participating in the program may start small and grow slowly. Creating a well-functioning ACO will require a significant investment of money, effort, and time and the traditional FFS program will still be an attractive alternative; particularly for providers who are accustomed to being rewarded for the volume of services they individually provide and are proficient at increasing volume. Therefore, it would be a mistake to assess the success of the shared savings program by counting how many ACOs participate in the initial agreement period. Making the ACO terms generous enough to lure a large number of ACOs into the program could mean a high percentage of ACOs failing to achieve savings for Medicare and also failing to deliver their patients high quality, coordinated care. It is not in the long-term interest of the shared savings program, or of Medicare more generally, to encourage participation by organizations that are unlikely to be successful. The program should not be expected to quickly transform the entire health-care delivery system. However, as a program that builds gradually, it could be an important step toward sustainability for the Medicare program if carefully designed to meet the goals of high quality care and slower growth in spending.

ACOs could play a central role in shifting the health care delivery system to one emphasizing quality and value to the benefit of the Medicare program, its beneficiaries, and taxpayers. However, the organization of care and care decisions will have to change if improvements are to be realized. Shifting from volume-driven to value-driven care will not be quick or easy, and it cannot be expected that a single set of regulations will be able to address all contingencies or difficulties that may arise. Therefore, it is crucial that the program be able to evolve and adapt over time. As ACOs gain experience with the program they may be able to provide guidance about what works and what does not to other ACOs and to organizations considering whether to join the program. CMS will need to make data available to the ACOs and entities such as MedPAC to help CMS determine the strengths and weaknesses of the different shared savings models and what aspects of the regulations may need to change. MedPAC also stands ready to help if technical clarifications or other legislative changes are needed. CMS should also take the opportunity to use the CMMI when that would be the most fruitful avenue to experiment with payment designs and move the program forward. The recently announced

Pioneer ACO demonstration should be helpful in this regard and is in keeping with the tenor of many of our comments on the shared savings program. Providing an opportunity for experimentation in at least the initial years of operation of the shared savings program is another approach that we discuss in our comments on the one-sided model and quality reporting.

ACOs represent an opportunity to transform the delivery system, but realizing that opportunity will require providers to change their practices and take a risk on a novel payment system and CMS to be flexible and responsive as the program evolves.

We use the terminology of the proposed rule where possible. Briefly, the key terms are: an agreement period for each ACO consists of three performance years. An initial spending benchmark is computed using three years of Medicare spending for the beneficiaries assigned to the ACO. Each year, an update amount is added to the prior year's benchmark to create a new benchmark for the performance year. That benchmark is then compared to actual Medicare spending to compute any savings or loss.

ASSIGNMENT OF BENEFICIARIES TO ACOS

The proposed rule asks for comments on whether beneficiaries should be assigned to ACOs prospectively, that is, before the performance year, or retrospectively, that is, after the performance year. It discusses arguments on both sides and comes down on the side of retrospective assignment because the evaluation of effectiveness will be on the population actually served while at the same time the ACO providers, not knowing for sure which beneficiaries are in their ACO, will treat all patients the same way. It also proposes sharing aggregate beneficiary level-data on those who would have been assigned in the benchmark period prior to performance measurement so that the ACO will have some idea of those who might be assigned to it in the performance period.

Comment

In any new Medicare program the rights and responsibilities of Medicare beneficiaries should be a primary consideration. Beneficiaries should know if their health care providers are operating under a new incentive structure. At the same time, for an ACO program to work well, beneficiaries will need to have greater engagement in their own care management. Properly structuring how the beneficiary is informed of his or her assignment to an ACO provider could help accomplish both of these goals but that will require prospective assignment. Prospective assignment will also improve adjustment for risk and quality reporting as we discuss in later sections of this letter.

Not informing beneficiaries would run the risk of a repeat of the managed care "backlash" experienced in the 1990s. The backlash resulted from patients feeling that they were being forced into managed care by their employers and that the financial benefits were accruing to employers health plans, or providers, not them. Some providers, many of whom were losing revenue due to managed care, were more than willing to feed patient concerns that the savings from managed care were being produced at the expense of the quality of care. This toxic combination of concerns resulted in the backlash: it behooves Medicare to pay close attention to patient notification so as not to repeat history.

Beneficiaries will have to be assigned prospectively if they are to be informed of their assignment to an ACO before care is delivered to them under that model. Prospective assignment uses claims data from a prior year to make the assignment. An ACO would first identify its primary care provider members to Medicare. Medicare would then assign beneficiaries to the ACO whose primary care had been provided in prior years by those members. The proposed rule argues that retrospective assignment is superior to prospective. Retrospective assignment would use data from the performance year to make the assignment. However, if retrospective assignment were used, neither the ACO nor the beneficiary would know at the beginning of that year who was assigned to the ACO and prior notification would be impossible.

We suggest that the beneficiaries be informed and, unless beneficiaries indicate otherwise, they remain in the ACO. If they decide that the change in incentives for their provider makes them too uncomfortable, Medicare should provide them some choice. One choice that the beneficiary always has is to switch from the assigned primary care provider to another provider who is not in an ACO. Another choice, some suggest, is to allow beneficiaries to stay with their providers who are in the ACO yet "opt out;" that is, not have their data count toward the ACO's performance. This differs from the option allowed beneficiaries in the proposed rule which only allows a beneficiary to decide whether their provider should be given their data and does not give the beneficiary the option to opt out of the ACO and stay with their primary care provider. On the one hand, the opt-out option we propose would give the beneficiaries more choice and allay worries they might have about the incentives in ACOs. On the other hand, allowing beneficiaries to opt out creates administrative complexity for CMS and an opportunity for the ACO to discourage participation by complex, costly beneficiaries who could harm the ACO's performance.

In our approach, beneficiaries would have to make an active decision to opt-out, otherwise, their data will be part of the ACO's evaluation. As has been seen in other programs such as assignment into Part B by the Social Security Administration (94 percent accept assignment), beneficiaries with a low-income subsidy into Part D drug plans, and private-sector employees into retirement plans, the opt-out approach preserves choice while preventing low take-up rates. A similar approach should be taken if CMS continues with retrospective assignment, essentially extending the data opt out mechanism in the proposed rule to include removing the beneficiary's data from the ACO's performance. If opting-out is allowed, an ACO's opt-out pattern should be examined annually. CMS should reconsider an ACO's participation if it is unable to retain a high percentage of its beneficiaries or if only beneficiaries with certain characteristics tend to opt-out.

Finally, notification should strengthen beneficiaries' engagement with their care management. Many think that patient engagement in programs such as home monitoring and shared decision making and in keeping their primary care provider informed will be essential for ACOs to succeed. Part of the notification process should inform beneficiaries of their opportunities and responsibilities to influence their own health and the health care coordination that the ACO is offering.

Risk Adjustment of the ACO Population

Risk adjustment in the Medicare program is designed to account for the effect that demographic characteristics and health status have on expected Medicare spending. The update amount in the shared savings program is proposed to be "the projected absolute amount of growth in per capita expenditures" [p. 19611]. This is essentially the expected growth in Medicare spending for a beneficiary with a risk score of 1.00, the national average risk score. Because it is using this amount as the update, the proposed rule needs to adjust an ACO's benchmark by its population's risk score to preserve equity among ACOs with populations that have different risk characteristics. That is, the update and the benchmark have to be consistent. The proposal uses the prospective HCC model to create risk scores for each beneficiary in each ACO as it does for each beneficiary in each MA plan.

The proposed rule sets the initial benchmark for an ACO according to the spending for the beneficiaries who would have been assigned (retrospectively) to that ACO in the three years preceding the agreement year adjusted for the average risk score of the assigned beneficiaries.[1]

The risk score is then not updated in the agreement years, rather the risk score for the initial benchmark panel is kept unchanged even if the beneficiary population changes. This approach eliminates the incentive for an ACO to optimize coding, that is, to report as many diagnoses as possible for its patients and hence increase their risk scores because, the risk score is calculated based in part on the number and severity of diagnoses. The Commission shares CMS's concerns regarding coding optimization and its effects, however, the Commission is also concerned that this approach creates incentives for the ACO providers to encourage expensive patients to seek care elsewhere and to avoid new expensive patients. It also disconnects the benchmark spending from the beneficiaries who are actually assigned to the ACO. CMS considers another option which would tie expected spending more closely to the assigned beneficiaries. However, CMS concludes that the additional adjustments needed in the second option would outweigh its benefits and propose using the first option described above. We propose a modified version of the second option below.

	Low	Medium	High
	Low cost/low risk patients little scope for near-term savings	High-cost/high-risk patients could benefit from care coordination	High cost/lower-risk patients could benefit from more efficient care
CMS incentive	Attract these patients	Discourage these patients from using ACO physicians	Discourage these patients from switching to ACO practice
Revised incentive	Neutral	Keep these patients	Recruit these patients

Figure 1. Potential for savings from ACO.

Comment

We suggest that expected spending should be tied to the assigned beneficiaries, and that incentives to avoid high-risk beneficiaries and optimize coding should be minimized to the extent possible. We describe an approach that does so later in this section. Figure 1 compares the incentives in the proposed rule with the incentives in the approach we suggest. It is important to remember that if ACOs are to save money for the program they will need to focus on patients who are high cost to the program. As shown in Figure 1, those high-cost patients can be either those who are high-cost and high-risk or those that are high-cost and lower-risk. We need incentives for ACOs to want to retain patients who are high-cost and high-risk because they can improve care coordination for those patients and thus reduce avoidable spending (e.g., preventable readmissions) and improve quality. We also want ACOs to have an incentive to recruit patients who are lower risk but have been high cost because they have been treated inefficiently by other providers.

The proposed rule incentives would encourage ACOs to avoid new patients who are expected to be high-cost patients, and possibly to make their practice less attractive to new patients with complex needs. Yet these are the patients who have the greatest potential for savings. CMS should consider an approach to risk adjustment that would create incentives to keep and recruit those very patients and allow the ACO to concentrate on patients with the greatest potential for savings, which would benefit both the program and the ACO. The approach should have four key objectives:

- Acknowledge differences in resource needs of patients treated by different ACOs.
- Create an incentive for the ACO to accept new complex patients who need care coordination and to continue to develop and maintain the capacity to treat those cases.
- Create an incentive to attract patients away from inefficient providers and those involved in inappropriate billing of services
- Minimize the effect of variations in coding intensity on payments.

The current method does not meet the first three objectives.

To meet these objectives, benchmark spending could be based on the assigned patients' historical spending and their individual historical risk score. Patients that have historically used more resources (risk adjusted) prior to the start of the three year agreement period would have higher benchmarks. New patients, those assigned in years two or three of the performance period, would bring their historical spending and risk scores with them. ACOs would have an incentive to serve patients with high benchmarks and attract new patients from inefficient providers because the high benchmark follows the patient. However, adjustments to the benchmark for continuing patients would change over time only to the same extent as the spending of a similar (i.e., similar age/gender/conditions) population of FFS beneficiaries at the national level would be expected to change.[2] ACOs would not be rewarded with a higher benchmark if their patients grow sicker faster than expected compared to national rates and will not be penalized if they keep their patients healthier than expected. In other words, additional coding of conditions over the three years will not affect payment. Coding optimization had a large effect on the savings calculation in the PGP demonstration and the Commission agrees with CMS that it is important that its effects be minimized in the shared savings program.

Benchmarks could be calculated prospectively if there were prospective assignment. Knowing their benchmark in advance would help the ACO to monitor its progress on spending. Some adjustment would need to be made at the end of the year for beneficiaries who move or join MA plans.

On balance, we think this approach would be more equitable because it would tie benchmarks more closely to the assigned beneficiaries; would give ACOs an incentive to do what they should do best, take care of more complex patients who would benefit the most from care coordination; and minimize the incentive to focus resources on coding optimization.

Quality Measurement and Scoring

In both the one-sided and two-sided risk models, the ACO's final sharing rate will be determined by how well the ACO performs on a set of quality measures, regardless of the amount of cost reduction. CMS proposes to use 65 quality measures across 5 domains of care to calculate an ACO's sharing rate. The 5 measure domains are:

- Patient/caregiver experience (7 measures)
- Care coordination (16 measures)
- Patient safety (2 measures)
- Preventive health (9 measures)
- At-risk populations/frail elderly health (31 measures)

CMS proposes that each measure would be weighted equally within a domain, and each domain would be weighted equally in calculating an ACO's total quality performance score.

In year 1 of the ACO's agreement period, CMS would only evaluate whether an ACO reported on all of the required quality measures; the ACO's actual performance on the measures would not be used in calculating the percentage of shared savings or penalties the ACO receives, only whether the ACO achieved 100 percent complete and accurate reporting on each measure. An ACO's actual performance on the measures would be used in years 2 and 3 of the agreement period. The ACO's performance on each measure for its assigned beneficiary population would be compared to FFS or MA national benchmarks if such exist for a given measure, or compared against an absolute percentage threshold (for example, 30 percent, 40 percent, 50 percent, etc.). If an ACO fails to meet the minimum performance standards in any domain, it has one year to improve its performance or its contract with CMS will be terminated. Failure to report on a quality measure or reporting inaccurate information also could result in contract termination.

The ACO's performance on each measure relative to the benchmark would be converted into a point score, ranging from 2 points for performance over the 90th percentile or 90 percent, stepping down in equal increments to zero points if the ACO's performance on a measure is below the 30th percentile of the MA or FFS benchmark or below 30 percent if there is no comparable benchmark.

The sum of these "quality points" would be used to calculate the score in each domain and then the domain scores would be averaged to determine the percentage of the available shared savings or losses the ACO would be awarded. For example, if there were 10 measures in a domain and an ACO achieved 18 quality points out of the total of 20 possible points (equal to 10 measures times the maximum of 2 points each), it would receive a 90 percent score for that domain. If it did the same for all domains it would receive 90 percent of the ACO's share of the available shared savings (for example, in the standard 2-sided risk model, this ACO would receive 90 percent of 60 percent of the shared savings, or 54 percent). This approach is referred to as the quality performance standard option.

Comment

The Commission appreciates the need for CMS to be vigilant in ensuring that providers participating in an ACO do not stint on clinically necessary care in response to the economic incentives inherent in the design of the shared savings program. However, providers are less likely to participate in the program if the costs of creating and maintaining an administrative structure to meet CMS's participation requirements are too high. We are concerned that the proposed quality measurement and reporting requirements would create an unnecessarily high barrier to providers' participation in the program, especially in the start-up stages of the program, and that the scoring method creates undue financial uncertainty.

Quality measurement

To simplify quality reporting we urge CMS to consider using a much more focused set of quality indicators that reflect the outcomes ACOs are designed to achieve: keeping the population healthy, better care coordination to reduce unnecessary and sometimes harmful spending, and better patient experience. To that end, we support most of the proposed health outcome and patient experience measures, but suggest that CMS significantly reduce the number of required clinical process measures (Table 1). The agency should also decrease the administrative burden of data reporting for the remaining process measures by using measures that can be calculated using claims data, at least for the first few years of program implementation. CMS could use a small number of claims-based measures that report rates at which the ACO provides clinically-indicated services to its patients with certain diagnoses prevalent among Medicare beneficiaries. This approach would be similar to that the Commission uses to annually evaluate the aggregate quality of physician and other ambulatory care services with the Medicare Ambulatory Care Indicators for the Elderly (MACIEs).[3] We have also recently discussed the feasibility of adapting some Healthcare Effectiveness Data and Information Set (HEDIS) measures that could be calculated using claims data, which is another option for CMS to consider for the ACO program.[4] We estimate that the number of measures could be reduced from 65 in the proposed rule to as few as 18 if only the proposed patient experience and outcome measures were used, or up to 40 if all of the proposed process measures that could be calculated using claims data also were included.

Table 1. Comments on Proposed Quality Measures by Quality Domain

Domain: Summary comments	Detailed comments
Patient/Caregiver Experience: Support as proposed	We support the use of the proposed measures from the Clinician/Group Consumer Assessment of Healthcare Providers and Systems (CAHPS) survey and the Medicare Advantage (MA) CAHPS survey. Patients may be more willing to stay assigned to the ACO if they know the provider's payments are dependent on patients' review of the quality of care provided. To complement the proposed ambulatory care and overall health status questions, CMS also may wish to consider adding an item from the Hospital CAHPS survey to measure the quality of the hospital patient experiences of ACO members, such as the "overall rating of hospital" question.
Care Coordination: Support with exceptions noted	We strongly support the proposed 30-day readmission rate, post-discharge physician visit and medication reconciliation measures, Care Transition Measure survey, and the AHRQ Prevention Quality Indicators (ambulatory care-sensitive condition admission rates).
30-day mortality rate: Add as complement to 30-day readmission rate	In addition to the proposed all-cause 30-day readmission rate, we urge CMS to add a parallel risk-adjusted all-cause 30-day post-discharge mortality rate. Using readmission rates alone may give an incomplete indication of the quality of care provided to beneficiaries during and in the critical transition period following an inpatient stay.
AHRQ admission rate measures: Analyze reliability with small sample sizes; use only reliable individual measures or combine into composite measure	For the AHRQ admission rate measures (PQIs), we observe that there may be very small sample sizes available for some of these measures in smaller ACOs and in all ACOs for a few of these measures, such as admissions for dehydration, which have relatively low prevalence and incidence across even the entire Medicare population. Very small sample sizes will decrease the statistical reliability of the measures and therefore increase the chance that observed differences in rates will be due to random variation. To address this problem, CMS could either drop the PQIs that have the least statistical reliability, combine the proposed PQIs into a composite "multiple-cause" ambulatory care sensitive admission rate measure, or

Table 1. (Continued)

Domain: Summary comments	Detailed comments
	use statistical techniques such as shrinkage estimation to increase the reliability of the measure.
Medicare EHR and e-Rx Incentive Program measures: Do not use	We do not support the proposed inclusion in this domain of five measures that would be based on the Medicare Electronic Health Record (EHR) and e-Prescribing Incentive programs. The individual physicians in an ACO already will have incentives through those two programs to become "meaningful users" of EHR systems and to use electronic prescribing for all of their Medicare patients, while including these measures in the shared savings program as well would discourage less technologically-sophisticated providers from attempting to implement an ACO. It may be challenging for an ACO to improve the quality and efficiency of care delivery without an interoperable EHR system, but the implementation of specific care delivery innovations should be decisions left to the providers who come together to form an ACO, with Medicare focused on measuring and publicly reporting the resulting improvements in health outcomes and cost growth reductions.
Patient Safety: Support, with exceptions noted below	The Commission is concerned about recently published studies indicating that rates of health-care acquired conditions (HACs) and other patient safety incidents remain unnecessarily high and that progress in improving patient safety has been slow.[5] We therefore support the inclusion of patient safety measures in the shared savings program with the exceptions noted below. The use of a composite measure for this domain is reasonable since the number of patient safety incidents in an ACO's covered population likely will be too small to yield statistically reliable results if these measures are calculated individually.
Serious reportable events: Include as proposed	The first five measures on the proposed list of HACs—foreign object retained after surgery; air embolism; blood incompatibility; pressure ulcer stages III and IV; and patient falls and traumaare—classified by the National Quality Forum as "serious reportable

Table 1. (Continued)

Domain: Summary comments	Detailed comments
	events" (SREs), formerly called "never events." To focus ACOs on the reduction and ultimately elimination of these patient safety events, we support the inclusion of these proposed measures, and urge CMS to expand the list to include additional SRE measures that have been endorsed by the National Quality Forum, such as patient death or serious injury associated with medication errors, and death or serious injury resulting from failure to follow up or communicate clinical information, as soon as practicable. Because the data for these measures would be collected from claims, including them would not increase the administrative burden on ACOs, but CMS would need to monitor the potential unintended consequences of creating a disincentive for providers to report SREs on claims.
Hospital-Acquired Infections: Use ongoing HAI reporting through CDC's National Healthcare Safety Network	CMS proposes to include three individual measures of hospital-acquired infections (HAIs) in the HAC composite measure: central line-associated bloodstream infection (CLABSI), catheter-associated urinary tract infection (CAUTI), and surgical site infection (SSI). CMS has already specified a CLABSI measure for hospitals that participate in the Medicare Hospital Inpatient Quality Reporting (IQR) Program (built on the reporting infrastructure of the CDC's National Healthcare Safety Network (NHSN)). CMS will include an NHSN-based SSI measure in the IQR Program in 2012 and has proposed to add a CAUTI measure in 2013. As CMS brings these measures on-line for use in the Hospital IQR Program, we urge CMS to use the same infrastructure for the collection and reporting of all three of these HAI rates for the shared savings program. Using claims data to calculate HAI rates, where there will be an incentive to under-report their occurrence, exacerbates the reliability problem. It would be more accurate and efficient to use the CDC/NHSN mechanism that CMS will implement over the next few years for these three types of HAIs.

Table 1. (Continued)

Domain: Summary comments	Detailed comments
Manifestations of poor glycemic control: Evaluate current clinical evidence underlying measure specifications, modify or delete as indicated	The proposed HAC measures include "Manifestations of Poor Glycem ic Control," which we are concerned may not meet our long-standing principle that CMS should use only widely-accepted, evidence-based measures for all Medicare quality-based payment and public reporting. Concerning this particular measure, research published within the last two years suggests that the use of clinical interventions to maintain glycemic control in some patients, especially the frail elderly, may adversely affect patient health outcomes.[6,7] We urge CMS to carefully consider the most recent clinical evidence on glycemic control for hospital inpatients and older patients with multiple comorbidities before deciding whether to use this measure.
AHRQ patient safety indicators composite: Do not use because of duplication of other HAC measures, statistical concerns	If the HAC measures discussed above are included in the HAC composite measure, it seems duplicative to also include the proposed AHRQ Patient Safety Indicator (PSI) composite measure. Several components of the proposed PSI composite measure overlap with the other HAC measures. ACO providers may find the individual or composite AHRQ PSI measures useful for internal quality improvement activities, but we are concerned with the statistical reliability of the AHRQ PSI measures in the context of affecting individual ACOs' bonuses or penalties.
Preventive Health and At-Risk Populations: Reduce number of measures and use only claims-based process measures for initial 3-year contract period	Illustrative examples of proposed measures that could be used consistent with our suggestion to use only claims-based process of care measures include the following: influenza immunization and pneumonia vaccination rates; breast and colorectal cancer screening rates; rate of cholesterol management of patients with cardiovascular conditions; rates of eye and foot examinations for patients diagnosed with diabetes; rate of left ventricular function testing for patients hospitalized withprincipal diagnosis of heart failure; prescription for certain kinds of drugs for patients with coronary artery disease.

When determining the final set of measures, CMS also should address the balance in the number of measures in each quality domain. If each domain score is weighted equally when they are averaged to compute an ACO's final percentage of available shared savings or losses, individual measures in effect will have more or less weight depending on the total number of measures in the domain. Individual measures in a domain with few total measures will have more weight in the quality score calculation, and vice versa. In the proposed rule, the number of measures in the domains ranges from 2 in patient safety to 31 in the at-risk populations domain. (However, of the two patient safety measures one is a composite of 10 individual measures, the other is a composite of eight measures—simple counts may be misleading.) If CMS reduces the total number of measures, we suggest that CMS also consider carefully balancing the number of measures across the domains to create an incentive for equal clinical focus across a parsimonious final set of measures.

After a period of initial implementation experience and learning by both the agency and ACOs, CMS could, if needed, add more complex measures, for example, intermediate outcome measures that require data from clinical records, such as laboratory test results, as ACOs deploy the health information technology and other administrative capabilities needed to efficiently and reliably capture and report clinical record-based measurement data. CMS could also retire some measures as outcome measures are refined and experience builds confidence in their use.

A few of the proposed measures would be based on hospital claims data (which CMS calculates) or data reported by hospitals through the CDC National Healthcare Safety Network (NHSN). We agree that these measures of hospital patient safety and hospital-acquired conditions should be included in the ACO quality measure to focus ACOs on reducing or eliminating these avoidable and clinically serious events for their patients. To minimize the administrative burden of reporting on these measures for small ACOs or those that do not include a hospital, CMS could leverage its existing quality measurement data, such as having all hospital-level measures be based on data already collected for the Hospital Inpatient Quality Reporting program for all of the hospital's Medicare patients. CMS then could compute a weighted average of the quality scores of the hospitals used by the ACO's patients to ensure that the ACO was admitting its patients to high quality hospitals. This approach would enable ACOs that do not include hospitals to report hospital measures easily, and it would avoid the small numbers problem that otherwise could occur when these measures of very rare events are computed solely on the basis of each ACO's admitted patients.

Quality scoring

CMS should simplify quality reporting and reduce uncertainty regarding the quality scoring. To reduce uncertainty, we suggest that CMS use a modified version of the quality threshold approach discussed in the proposed rule. As the rule states:

> "A threshold established at a basic level of quality acknowledged to be minimally necessary presents less of a risk of being triggered due to random variation, as opposed to truly poor performance. Finally, for ACOs meeting the threshold, their shared savings percentage attributable to quality would be fixed and certain. This would increase incentives, achieve savings, and present more certainty on potential investment returns for organizations considering whether or not to become ACOs." [P.19597-8]

We agree with this logic and find that the advantages of the quality threshold option (compared with the proposed quality performance standard option) would outweigh any disadvantages cited, particularly in the early years of the program.

A threshold approach could work as follows. First, CMS could tell each ACO what the historical 50th percentile has been for each quality metric in prior years. The ACO then would have to exceed this benchmark in each of the five domains to fully share in savings. For each domain in which it exceeded the benchmark, its share of savings would increase by 20 percent of the maximum shared savings percentage. This would give the ACO certainty over the targets it needs to achieve and reduce the uncertainty over its financial liability, which plagues the proposed quality approach. Whatever the ACO score on the quality metrics, the ACO is still responsible for its share of losses under the two-sided model. The proposed rule sets the loss sharing at one minus the actual savings share. That design can lead to asymmetries in the model. For example, if the quality score were 40 percent and the maximum shared savings rate were 60 percent, the share of savings would be the product, 24 percent. The share of loss would be one minus the share of savings, or 76 percent. The Pioneer ACO demonstration also recognizes this asymmetry as an issue. Our alternative design would set the share of losses equal to the maximum sharing rate because that would reduce uncertainty and the expectation would be that ACOs will likely be above average on all five domains most of the time.

Assessing Benchmarks, Spending and Savings at Standardized Prices

The proposed rule asks for comment on whether or not to take into account factors such as the Medicare wage index and teaching payments to hospitals when calculating benchmarks, spending, and savings (or losses). The proposed rule does not take these factors into account primarily because the statute states that benchmarks "...shall be adjusted for beneficiary characteristics and such other factors as the Secretary determines appropriate..." but the only adjustment specified for the expenditures used in the savings calculation is "...for beneficiary characteristics,..." The proposed rule concludes that the Secretary does not have authority to adjust expenditures for other factors.

Comment

We suggest that two underlying principles should be kept in mind when considering this issue. First, the benchmark, expenditures, and update should all be consistent to the extent possible. Second, ACOs should primarily be judged on their success in controlling the growth in service use by their patients isolated from changes in prices (such as input prices in their markets) that may be outside of the ACOs control. Maintaining these two principles will be crucial to create a shared savings program that is equitable for ACOs in different parts of the country and that use different mixes of providers. Given the importance of this calculation, we think it is critical that CMS reexamine whether it has the authority to follow these principles and if it determines it does not, CMS should seek a statutory change that would grant the agency this authority; and MedPAC will also pursue this legislative change.

To the first principle, because the update is specified as the projected absolute increase in national per capita spending, the benchmark and spending should be standardized so that they will be consistent with the update. For example the update essentially incorporates the national average wage index, GPCI, and other geographic price adjusters. Standardizing ACO spending for those geographic adjusters would be equitable because it would remove any advantage or disadvantage from an event outside the ACO's control, namely the input price for labor in their region. Similarly, Medicare makes adjustment for additional products such as teaching through the IME factor, technology adoption through special DRG adjustments, and other policy goals such as access in rural areas through factors such as special payments to CAHs. Standardizing for these policy factors would be more equitable as well because those special payments are not for the service provided but to achieve other policy goals—which we would not want to discourage ACOs from achieving. The method used to standardize ACO spending could follow that laid out in our recent report on geographic variation.[8]

To the second principle, concentrating on service use, two examples may indicate why adjusting for prices is important. For example, assume a group practice operates in an area where the hospital has a wage index exception. The exception expires, and then hospital payments fall by 8 percent. This should not be a reason for the group practice to receive a bonus. Likewise, imagine a group of physicians operating in a rural area served by a midsize hospital and two small hospitals. The small hospitals convert to CAH status and that allows the midsize hospital to convert to sole community hospital status and hospital payments go up by 10 percent. That should not be a reason to assess the group with a penalty. To avoid allowing idiosyncrasies and fluctuation in prices over time to affect bonuses and penalties, the ACO program should make adjustments for input prices and special payments.

USING HISTORICAL SERVICE USE TO ADJUST THE MAXIMUM SAVINGS RATE

Once the level of service use is computed, it might then be more equitable to adjust the rewards for ACOs that have already achieved relatively low service use levels. One approach could be to allow such ACOs to obtain a larger share of the savings by increasing the maximum savings rate for ACOs with the lowest service use. Those ACOs could for example, have a maximum savings rate of 75 percent in the one-sided model or 95 percent in the two-sided model. ACOs with higher baseline service use would have a lower maximum savings rate. This approach would recognize that ACOs with lower service use may have less scope for efficiency gains than other ACOs and thus, increasing their share of savings might help increase equity across ACOs.

ASSIGNMENT BASED ON ONLY PRIMARY CARE SERVICES PROVIDED BY A PRIMARY CARE PHYSICIAN

Under the proposed rule assignment is based on the primary care physicians who account for the plurality of primary care charges, and the primary care physician has to be exclusive to one ACO. Assignment is not extended to specialist physicians or to non-physician practitioners such as nurse practitioners, advanced practice nurses, or physician assistants. Rural health clinics and FQHCs are also not used for assignment. To encourage use of FQHCs and RHCs, CMS increases the percentage of savings ACOs can get based on percent of assigned beneficiaries with one visit or more to an FQHC or RHC in the ACO and reduces the additional threshold in the one-sided model on a similar basis.

Comment

CMS points out that the statute specifies that assignment be based on "...utilization of primary care services provided under this title by an ACO professional described in subsection (h)(1)(A)." An ACO professional described in (h)(1) could be either a physician or a practitioner, but (h)(1)(A) refers to physicians only. In addition to restricting assignment to physicians, the proposed rule further restricts assignment to primary care physicians because it would be consistent with other provisions in PPACA and because it "... places priority on the services of designated primary care physicians (for example, internal medicine, general practice, family practice, and geriatric medicine) in the assignment process." The Pioneer ACO demonstration explicitly adds nurse practitioners and physician assistants to the definition of primary care provider. It also creates a second step in the assignment algorithm allowing beneficiaries to be assigned to specialist physicians under certain circumstances. A step-wise option is also discussed in the proposed rule but is not the preferred option because it would increase complexity and require specialist to be exclusive to one ACO, even though it might increase the number of beneficiaries assigned.

The Commission prefers a more expansive definition of providers who could be assigned beneficiaries to increase the number of beneficiaries assigned to ACOs and to recognize the role those providers play in patient care. For example, we would prefer the step-wise option which assigns beneficiaries first to primary care physicians if possible and then to certain specialty physicians if the share of evaluation and management visits (or charges) to primary care physicians falls below a threshold value.[9] (The Pioneer ACO demonstration sets the threshold as 10 percent or less of E&M charges.) Although those specialists would have to be exclusive to one ACO for assignment purposes, they could still serve other patients who are either not assigned to ACOs or are assigned to other ACOs, thus the assignment exclusivity should not create access problems. The question of whether beneficiaries can be assigned to other practitioners should also be considered. Here again the Commission would urge CMS to reexamine its legislative authority, and if it determines that it is unable to pursue the broader definition for assignment, the agency should seek legislative clarification or the requisite authority and MedPAC will seek legislation as well.

It would also be more straightforward to allow assignment of patients to RHCs and FQHCs and encourage their use directly rather than to introduce special provisions for the savings share and thresholds as the proposed rule does. These are primary care provider teams often associated with a physician and usually providing primary care services. Logically they should be allowed to participate in ACOs and patients should be assigned to them. In many rural areas, RHCs function as primary care physicians' offices and, although they are paid differently under Medicare, they are still fulfilling the same function. In addition, under the proposed rule, beneficiaries could not be assigned to an ACO if they received all of their primary care services from RHCs. If many of the beneficiaries in an area were in this situation it would make it difficult to establish ACOs in such areas. A similar problem could be true in areas where many patients are seen by FQHCs. The proposed rule points out that an additional obstacle to assignment is that services in RHCs and FQHCs are generally paid on a flat rate and their claim do not specify whether they are for primary care services or not. We propose CMS posit that all claims in RHCs and FQHCs are for primary care services and use them for assignment as it would any other primary care claim.

SINGLE-SIDED SHARED SAVINGS MODEL

In the proposed rule a single-sided shared savings model is discussed that will last for two years and then transition to a two-sided model. It notes that a strictly one-sided model "...may not be enough of an incentive for participants to improve the efficiency of health care delivery and cost." The "hybrid approach" proposed is expected to allow organization to gain experience with population management before assuming risk. More experienced organization can choose to enter directly into a two-sided risk model that allows ACOs a greater share of savings in recognition of the greater risk that they accept.

Comment

Although the hybrid approach is reasonable in terms of moving to a program with stronger incentives for improving care, it may occur too soon for organizations that are uncertain of success. One possibility would be to give ACOs a choice to remain in the one-sided model through the three years of the first agreement period. Forcing ACOs to make too quick a transition could increase the risk of failure, and reduce participation. During those first years, CMS could analyze the data on performance and report on how the ACOs would have fared under a two-sided model and under different values for the savings percentage and other key parameters. CMS could also report on observed variation and use information on early adopters to inform subsequent regulations. Those follow-on regulations might make other models available and modify specifications for savings percentages and thresholds. This might make entry more feasible for ACOs with different characteristics than those in the early years as the parameters for success become more apparent.

To protect the taxpayer, if the one-sided model is extended, CMS would need to maintain the proposed minimum savings rates (MSR). Even with the currently proposed minimum saving rates and bonus thresholds there will still be some bonuses paid for random variation. The MSR and threshold are needed to limit the size of bonuses paid for random variation, and thus limit the risk of ACOs increasing Medicare costs. When offering the one-sided and two-sided models at the same time, CMS should also continue to assure that the two sided model is relatively attractive, recognizing that ACOs are taking some risk in that model. The share of savings and other variables should be designed to take that into account.

While the time frame of the one-sided model should be extended beyond two years, the two sided model should be retained as an option and eventually should be the only option. Given the proposed rules, providers who have confidence that they can generate an annual one percent reduction in the growth rate of Medicare expenditures (cumulatively, three percent over the three year agreement period) will be better off under the two sided model rather than the one sided model. The Medicare program would also benefit from the stronger incentives to change practice patterns inherent in the two-sided model.

IMPROVING THE RETURN ON INVESTMENT FOR ACO FORMATION

When deciding whether to form ACOs, providers will weigh the prospect of bonuses against the costs of forming an ACO. Changing the ACO regulations to reduce the fixed costs of forming and operating an ACO will be necessary to attract providers to the ACO model. This will be particularly important for small ACOs. At the same time, increasing the share of savings going to providers beyond the maximum of 50 percent for the one-sided shared savings model or 60 percent for the two-sided shared savings model would improve the benefit side of the equation. For example, for the first agreement period the savings rate could be up to 75 percent for the one-sided model and 95 percent for the two-sided model. (CMS would need to retain the minimum savings rate and the thresholds to limit the cost of paying bonuses for random variation.)

The proposed rule already has two provisions that favor smaller ACOs without hospitals. First, small ACOs without a hospital have less stringent minimum saving rates (MSRs), allowing them a 10 percent chance of receiving a random bonus compared to a 1 percent chance for the largest ACOs. Second, under the bonus-only shared savings model, small ACOs with certain characteristics (such as only ACO professionals—no hospital) receive a share of first dollar savings if they meet their MSR, while large ACOs and those with hospitals receive a share of savings net of the first 2 percent of savings. For example a physician-only ACO with 5,000 beneficiaries that generates a 4% reduction in Medicare cost growth over two years would be eligible for up to a 2% bonus (50% of 4%) while the same ACO with a hospital partner or a larger ACO would only receive up to 1% bonus (50% x (4% - 2%). Therefore, the bonus structure is already set up to favor small ACOs.

What will prevent small ACOs from joining under the proposed rule (and may prevent larger providers from joining also) are the high fixed costs of forming and operating an ACO. To that end, the final rule could:

- Shift quality reporting to metrics that can be measured with claims and hospital-reported data as discussed above.
- Reduce administrative requirements of forming the ACO, such as having CMS compute market share statistics to free ACOs from the administrative burden of evaluating their own compliance with the FTC safe harbors.
- Eliminate criteria concerned with the process of how an ACO operates such as requirements on board composition, method of distributing savings among ACO participants, and meaningful use of electronic medical records.

The general idea is that bending the Medicare cost trend downward is difficult, and thus ACOs will have to change practice patterns to succeed, and even then may have limited opportunities for savings in most markets in the near term. To make entrance into the shared savings program economically attractive for these providers, CMS should set a goal of keeping the annual administrative costs of operating ACO to less than one percent of Medicare expenditures per beneficiary. For an ACO with 5,000 beneficiaries this would be roughly $500,000. In other words, the marginal cost of adding an ACO to a group practice should be less than $500,000 additional dollars beyond what is currently spent on administration and compliance with other requirements such as PQRI and HIT. This would allow a high-quality ACO that generates two percent savings to receive more in bonuses than the cost of operating the ACO. While CMS should try to reduce administrative burdens on ACOs, CMS needs to maintain the MSR at its current level to prevent excessive bonus payments due to random variation in ACO spending. In other words, CMS should make ACOs more attractive by reducing the cost of forming ACOs rather than lowering the thresholds that providers must achieve to share in savings.

One principle that should be followed is to focus on outcomes and not process for all aspects of the program, not just quality metrics. For example, we are interested in ACOs that work; not how their internal structure brings success about. Decisions on the structure of board membership and distributing savings bonuses within the ACO should be left to their discretion, not directed by regulation. Removing regulation that focus on internal processes within ACOs would simplify the regulation and decrease the costs of forming ACOs.

CONCLUSION

Taken together, a number of our comments should make the ACO shared savings program more attractive to smaller, physician led ACOs including those with no hospital participation. Streamlining quality reporting, particularly for hospital measures, should limit administrative burden on ACOs. Extending the one-sided model should remove the fear of having an unknown liability for the ACO participants. Allowing assignment to RHCs and FQHCs might make physician led ACOs more feasible in areas served by those providers. CMS could also coordinate with other agencies such as the FTC to reduce administrative burden on ACOs. Many of these steps could make forming ACOs a less capital-intensive process, which would remove a barrier for smaller, physician-led organizations. Finally, CMS could also consider creating demonstration of smaller, physician-led ACOs through the CMMI.

To increase the attractiveness of the ACO program to providers, CMS could reduce the costs of forming an ACO and could increase the share of savings going to providers beyond the current maximum of 50 percent for a one-sided shared savings model or 60 percent for the two-side risk sharing model. For example, for the first agreement period the savings rate could be up to 75 percent for the one-sided model and 95 percent for the two-sided model. However, CMS needs to retain the minimum savings rate and the thresholds to limit the cost of paying bonuses for random variation.

MedPAC appreciates your consideration of these policy issues. Thoughtful and effective regulations and demonstration designs will be necessary for ACOs to succeed. The Commission also values the ongoing cooperation and collaboration between CMS and MedPAC staff on technical policy issues. We look forward to continuing this productive relationship.

If you have any questions, or require clarification of these issues, please feel free to contact Mark Miller, MedPAC's Executive Director, at 202-220-3700.

Sincerely,

Glenn M. Hackbarth
Chairman

End Notes

1 The actual calculation is more complicated including truncation of unusually high spending for an individual beneficiary, weighting by year, and other adjustments.

2 Under this approach, using the claims history of each beneficiary assigned to the ACO, one could use the variables in the HCC calculation to characterize each beneficiary in the ACO and match them to similar beneficiaries in the overall FFS population. Let us call that set of similar beneficiaries group R. One could then compute how the spending for group R has grown historically compared to average spending growth in the overall FFS population. This differential growth rate would be the amount allowed beyond the update for beneficiaries in the ACO with characteristics similar to group R. Because the assignment to group R is based on the beneficiary's historical spending and claims it would not change due to coding changes in the performance period. Technically, the differential growth rate, plus one, multiplied by the beneficiary's prior benchmark, added to the update, would yield the beneficiary's new benchmark. The ACO's benchmark would be the average of its beneficiaries' benchmarks.

Conceptually, this approach is similar to that proposed for the Pioneer ACO demonstration. In both cases the goal is to make the update consistent with the benchmark and only allow for growth in spending similar to the growth observed in a matched cohort of the national FFS population. (This is different from the PGP demonstration in which target spending was based on the concurrent performance of a comparison group drawn from the local area. Instead, benchmarks would be based on historical cost growth of similar patients in the national FFS population, not a local comparison group.) In the Pioneer ACO demonstration, the adjustment is made to the update. In the shared savings program, because the update is specified in statute, the adjustment has to be made to the benchmark.

3 *Report to the Congress: Medicare payment policy.* MedPAC, March 2011.

4 *Report to the Congress: Medicare payment policy.* MedPAC, March 2010.

5 MedPAC comment letter on proposed rule for Medicare Hospital Value-Based Purchasing Program, March 4, 2011.

6 Montori, V. M. and M. Fernández-Balsells. 2009. Glycemic control in type 2 diabetes: Time for an evidence-based about-face? *Annals of Internal Medicine* 150, no. 11 (June 2): 803-808.

7 Lee, S. J. and C. Eng. 2011. Goals of glycemic control in frail older patients with diabetes. *Journal of the American Medical Association* 305, no. 13 (April 6): 1350–1351.

8 *Report to the Congress: Regional variation in Medicare service use.* MedPAC, January 2011.

9 Assignment is to the group of primary care physicians in the ACO or the group of specialists in the ACO, not at the individual physician level.

CHAPTER SOURCES

Chapter 1 – This is an edited, reformatted and augmented version of Congressional Research Service Report R41474, dated May 26, 2011.

Chapter 2 – This website information has been edited, reformatted and augmented from www.medpac.gov/.../06062011_ACO_CMS1345_ MedPAC_COMMENT.pdf

INDEX

A

Accountable Care Organizations (ACOs), 1, iii, v, vii, 1, 2, 3, 4, 5, 6, 7, 8, 9, 10, 11, 12, 13, 14, 15, 16, 18, 19, 20, 21, 22, 23, 24, 25, 26, 27, 29, 30, 31, 34, 35, 36, 37, 38, 40, 41, 42, 43, 44, 45, 46, 47, 48, 49, 50, 51, 52, 54, 56, 57, 58, 59, 60, 61, 62, 63, 65, 66, 67, 68, 70, 72,73, 75, 76, 78, 79, 80, 81, 82, 83, 84, 85, 86, 87, 88, 89
agencies, 24, 25, 46, 66, 89
air embolism, 77
algorithm, 54, 84
American Recovery and Reinvestment Act, 10, 61
antitrust, 2, 3, 24, 32, 46, 47, 48, 49, 50, 59, 62, 66
asymmetry, 81
at-risk populations, 80
authority, 16, 20, 22, 28, 82, 85

B

backlash, 69
base, 23, 31
benchmarks, 8, 66, 72, 73, 74, 82, 90
beneficiaries, viii, 2, 8, 11, 12, 13, 15, 16, 17, 18, 19, 22, 23, 26, 27, 28, 29, 30, 31, 32, 33, 34, 35, 36, 37, 41, 42, 46, 47, 52, 53, 54, 55, 59, 60, 62, 66, 67, 68, 69, 70, 71, 72, 73, 75, 76, 84, 85, 87, 88, 90
benefits, 21, 47, 49, 50, 69, 71
board members, 88
bonuses, 4, 8, 25, 79, 83, 86, 87, 88, 89

C

CAP, 29, 32
capital expenditure, 61
category a, 50
catheter, 78
CBS, 58
CDC, 78, 80
Centers for Medicare and Medicaid Services (CMS), vii, 2, 8, 23, 24, 25, 26, 27, 28, 29, 30, 31, 32, 33, 34, 35, 36, 37, 38, 39, 41, 43, 44, 45, 46, 47, 49, 50, 51, 54, 55, 58, 60, 61, 62, 65, 66, 67, 68, 70, 71, 72, 73, 74, 75, 76, 78, 79, 80, 81, 82, 84, 85, 86, 87, 88, 89
certification, 28
cholesterol, 79
clinical interventions, 79
coding, 71, 72, 73, 90
colorectal cancer, 79
community, 5, 9, 13, 17, 20, 83
compensation, 60
compliance, 13, 23, 27, 32, 88
confidentiality, 30

Congress, iv, 58, 61, 90
Congressional Budget Office, 2, 9, 58, 59, 61
consensus, 9
consumer choice, 50
consumers, 15, 21, 46, 47
coordination, 13, 29, 31, 39, 66, 70, 71, 72, 73, 75
coronary artery disease, 79
cost, viii, 2, 4, 5, 6, 7, 11, 12, 13, 14, 15, 17, 18, 20, 21, 23, 25, 26, 47, 58, 59, 62, 66, 71, 72, 73, 77, 85, 87, 88, 89, 90
cost saving, 5, 14, 21
counsel, 10

D

data set, 31
dehydration, 76
demographic characteristics, 70
demonstrations, 8, 57
Department of Health and Human Services, 2, 3, 24
Department of Justice, 2, 24, 46
diabetes, 79, 90
diseases, 13
distribution, 24, 32, 46
doctors, 14, 20, 60
DOJ, 46, 47, 48, 49, 50, 54
drugs, 79

E

earnings, 14
economic incentives, 75
economies of scale, 14
emergency, 14
employees, 5, 17, 57, 70
employers, 69
employment relationship, 14
enforcement, 46
enrollment, 23
equipment, 14, 25
equity, 70, 83

evidence, 17, 18, 26, 47, 49, 66, 79, 90
examinations, 79
exercise, 30, 31
expenditures, 2, 8, 10, 12, 18, 21, 35, 36, 37, 38, 42, 43, 46, 52, 59, 61, 82, 86, 88

F

federal criminal law, 28
Federal Register, viii, 61, 62, 65
fee-for-service (FFS), viii, 5, 12, 16, 17, 18, 20, 21, 28, 35, 36, 37, 38, 39, 46, 52, 53, 66, 67, 73, 74, 90
financial, vii, 1, 2, 3, 6, 8, 13, 18, 20, 22, 24, 27, 32, 34, 47, 54, 69, 75, 81
financial incentives, vii, 1, 3, 6, 8, 24, 27
financial reports, 54
fixed costs, 87
formation, 2, 5, 16, 48, 50
formula, 11, 12, 42, 43, 44, 62
Fragmented care, vii, 1, 3
fraud, 54
free choice, 31
funding, 46
funds, 10, 41, 46

G

goods and services, 14
governance, 16, 17, 20, 48, 54
growth, viii, 4, 12, 18, 22, 25, 35, 36, 46, 52, 61, 66, 67, 70, 77, 82, 86, 87, 90
growth rate, 86, 90
guidance, 44, 46, 47, 54, 67
guidelines, 13

H

harbors, 88
HCC, 35, 52, 62, 71, 90
health, vii, 1, 2, 3, 4, 5, 6, 7, 8, 9, 10, 11, 12, 14, 17, 19, 20, 21, 22, 24, 25, 29, 30, 31, 34, 35, 36, 39, 46, 47, 50, 51, 55, 56, 57,

59, 60, 61, 67, 68, 69, 70, 73, 75, 76, 77, 79, 80, 84, 85
Health and Human Services, vii, 1, 3
health care, vii, 1, 2, 3, 4, 5, 7, 8, 9, 10, 11, 14, 17, 19, 20, 21, 22, 24, 29, 31, 46, 47, 50, 51, 56, 59, 60, 61, 67, 68, 70, 85
health care costs, 11, 29
health care professionals, 24
health care system, 3, 14, 19, 21, 56
health information, 10, 23, 30, 31, 61, 80
health insurance, 29, 31
health status, 11, 12, 29, 35, 36, 70, 76
heart failure, 59, 79
HHS, 2, 3, 24, 55
history, 7, 69, 90
hospitalization, 16, 59
House, 60, 61
House of Representatives, 61
hybrid, 52, 57, 85, 86
hypertension, 57

I

immunization, 79
improvements, 4, 8, 10, 13, 23, 67, 77
income, 70
individuals, 3, 9, 11, 15, 19, 24, 29, 31, 46
industry, 46
infection, 78
influenza, 79
infrastructure, 6, 16, 25, 45, 78
injury, 78
integrated care delivery model in Medicare, vii, 1, 3
integration, 10, 19, 47, 48
internal processes, 88
Internal Revenue Service, 2, 24
investment(s), 10, 16, 19, 25, 58, 67, 81
issues, viii, 2, 3, 15, 24, 54, 59, 65, 66, 89

J

joint ventures, 9, 17, 57, 61

L

laws, 32, 46, 47, 49, 50, 54, 62
lead, 8, 10, 21, 81
leadership, 6, 17, 44, 47, 48, 66
learning, 58, 80
legislation, 61, 85
legislative authority, 85
loans, 58
low risk, 71
lower prices, 47

M

management, viii, 7, 13, 17, 29, 47, 54, 66, 69, 70, 79, 85, 86
market concentration, 2
market position, 10
market share, 88
marketing, 31, 32, 58
measurement, 56, 75, 80
media, 56, 57
median, 45
Medicaid, vii, 2, 4, 6, 7, 8, 11, 13, 45, 51, 56, 59, 60, 65
medical, 4, 6, 7, 8, 9, 10, 11, 12, 14, 16, 18, 19, 25, 33, 57, 58, 61, 62, 88
medical care, 6, 11, 14, 19, 58
Medicare, v, vii, 1, 2, 3, 4, 7, 8, 11, 12, 13, 15, 16, 17, 18, 19, 20, 21, 22, 23, 24, 25, 26, 27, 28, 29, 30, 31, 32, 33, 34, 35, 36, 37, 38, 39, 41, 42, 43, 44, 45, 46, 47, 48, 49, 50, 51, 52, 53, 54, 55, 56, 58, 59, 60, 61, 62, 65, 66, 67, 68, 69, 70, 75, 76, 77, 78, 79, 80, 82, 85, 86, 87, 88, 90
Medicare Payment Advisory Commission (MedPAC), v, vii, 9, 22, 26, 58, 59, 61, 62, 65, 67, 82, 85, 89, 90, 91
Medicare Shared Savings Program, v, vii, 1, 2, 3, 16, 21, 25, 36, 45, 46, 47, 48, 49, 50, 51, 52, 53, 54, 55, 59, 61, 62, 65
medication, 19, 76, 78
medicine, 17, 26, 47, 54, 58, 84
membership, 54

methodology, 62
MMA, 8
models, vii, 1, 3, 5, 10, 12, 14, 15, 17, 18, 19, 20, 21, 34, 41, 51, 54, 56, 57, 58, 63, 66, 67, 73, 86
mortality rate, 76
multiple unrelated providers, vii, 1, 3

N

negotiating, 21, 24
nucleus, 7
nurses, 84

O

obstacles, 20
Office of the Inspector General, 2, 24
operations, 32
opportunities, 70, 88
opt out, 53, 69, 70
optimization, 71, 73
overlap, 66, 79

P

participants, 9, 10, 24, 26, 27, 28, 29, 31, 32, 34, 42, 44, 46, 47, 48, 49, 50, 54, 62, 85, 88, 89
patient care, 66, 84
Patient Protection and Affordable Care Act, vii, viii, 1, 3, 46, 65
Patient Protection and Affordable Care Act (PPACA), vii, viii, 1, 2, 3, 5, 7, 16, 18, 21, 25, 26, 27, 45, 46, 47, 51, 56, 57, 59, 60, 61, 65, 84
PCP, 54
penalties, 2, 24, 28, 30, 32, 74, 79, 83
per capita cost, 40
per capita expenditure, 18, 35, 36, 41, 52, 70
percentile, 39, 45, 74, 81
performance measurement, 68
physical therapist, 24

physicians, vii, 1, 4, 5, 6, 7, 9, 10, 11, 12, 15, 16, 17, 20, 21, 22, 24, 25, 26, 28, 33, 34, 48, 50, 54, 57, 58, 59, 62, 71, 77, 83, 84, 85, 90
pneumonia, 79
policy, 2, 20, 24, 46, 57, 63, 83, 89, 90
policy issues, 89
poor performance, 56, 81
population, 2, 4, 6, 8, 11, 12, 13, 20, 25, 29, 30, 32, 36, 39, 51, 52, 53, 57, 58, 66, 68, 70, 71, 73, 74, 75, 76, 77, 86, 90
principles, 46, 54, 82
professionals, 7, 16, 27, 36, 57, 62, 87
profit, 5
proposed regulations, 3, 26, 27, 30, 45
protection, 31
provider payments, vii, 1, 3

Q

qualifications, 66
quality improvement, 6, 13, 23, 79

R

recognition, 4, 40, 86
recommendations, iv
reconciliation, 41, 76
Reform, 58, 60, 61
regulations, 28, 32, 46, 47, 49, 51, 55, 58, 59, 60, 67, 86, 87, 89
regulatory changes, 32
regulatory requirements, 30
rehabilitation, 25
reinsurance, 41
reliability, 76, 77, 78, 79
requirements, 13, 16, 30, 32, 37, 40, 42, 43, 44, 45, 50, 53, 54, 75, 88
resolution, 32
resources, 6, 33, 72, 73
response, 62, 75
restrictions, 45
retirement, 70
revenue, 69

rewards, 7, 67, 83
rights, iv, 68
risk(s), viii, 12, 18, 19, 21, 29, 32, 35, 39, 40, 48, 52, 59, 61, 62, 66, 67, 68, 69, 70, 71, 72, 73, 74, 76, 81, 86, 89
rules, 32, 47, 54, 86
rural areas, 6, 9, 83, 85

S

safety, 39, 48, 49, 50, 73, 77, 78, 79, 80
sanctions, 30
savings, viii, 2, 4, 5, 8, 10, 11, 12, 13, 14, 15, 16, 17, 18, 22, 24, 27, 28, 29, 32, 33, 34, 35, 36, 37, 38, 40, 41, 42, 43, 44, 45, 46, 47, 51, 52, 55, 58, 59, 60, 61, 62, 65, 66, 67, 68, 69, 70, 71, 72, 73, 74, 75, 77, 78, 80, 81, 82, 83, 84, 85, 86, 87, 88, 89, 90
savings rate, 11, 36, 37, 42, 81, 83, 86, 87, 89
scope, 59, 71, 83
Senate, 60
service provider, 48
services, iv, vii, 1, 3, 4, 7, 8, 10, 12, 13, 15, 16, 17, 18, 20, 21, 25, 26, 27, 28, 29, 31, 32, 33, 35, 36, 37, 47, 50, 52, 54, 57, 58, 60, 62, 67, 72, 75, 84, 85
signs, 31
Social Security, 25, 36, 70
Social Security Administration, 70
specialists, 7, 9, 13, 14, 15, 17, 20, 22, 24, 27, 54, 55, 57, 62, 85, 90
specifications, 45, 79, 86
spending, viii, 2, 4, 12, 18, 22, 25, 41, 42, 54, 66, 67, 68, 70, 71, 72, 73, 75, 82, 88, 90
SSI, 78
stakeholders, 2, 19, 25, 55
state, 6, 26, 53, 56
states, 81, 82
statistics, 88
structure, 14, 17, 20, 22, 24, 26, 37, 46, 47, 48, 54, 59, 66, 68, 75, 87, 88

structuring, 69
subsidy, 70
supplier, 28, 30, 32, 33
suppliers, 16, 17, 20, 25, 27, 29, 31, 32, 33, 58
sustainability, 67

T

target, 12, 34, 90
taxpayers, 67
teams, 85
techniques, 77
technology, 10, 23, 34, 55, 61, 80, 83
tension, 23
testing, 19, 79
time frame, 86
total costs, 8
total revenue, 51
trade, 46
transition period, 76
treatment, 8, 14, 46, 47, 48
Trust Fund, 41
type 2 diabetes, 90

U

ulcer, 77
urban areas, 8
urinary tract infection, 78

V

variables, 86, 90
variations, 72

W

waiver, 54
Washington, 56, 57, 58, 59, 60, 61, 62, 65
wellness, 26